calorie
counter

Dr Wynnie Chan

hamlyn

Nutrient information has been calculated using data from the UK Food Nutrient Databank which is available from The Food Standards Agency (FSA). Some values have been estimated based on similar foods. The information in this book is intended only as a guide to following a healthy diet. People with special dietary requirements of any kind should consult appropriate medical professionals before changing their diet.

An Hachette Livre UK Company

www.hachettelivre.co.uk

First published in Great Britain in 2003 by Hamlyn,

a division of Octopus Publishing Group Ltd,

2–4 Heron Quays, London E14 4JP

www.octopusbooks.co.uk

This edition published in 2009

Copyright © Octopus Publishing Group Ltd 2003, 2009

This material was previously published as Food & Diet Counter

ISBN 978-0-600-61920-8

A CIP catalogue record for this book is available from the British Library

Printed and bound in China

10 9 8 7 6 5 4 3 2 1

CONTENTS

Whether you want to lose just a few kilograms or rather more, eating healthily is vital. This does not mean cutting out all of your favourite treats completely, just eating them in moderation. If you're not enjoying your food, you are less likely to stick to your diet and exercise regime.

Losing weight doesn't just mean that you'll have more energy and feel better about yourself, it also decreases the risk of developing various ailments, including diabetes, hypertension, coronary heart disease, stroke, respiratory problems, gallstones and some cancers.

What is a healthy weight?

The formula used to establish whether a person is too thin, the right weight, fat or obese is called the Body Mass Index (BMI). This is a simple measurement of weight against height, and can be calculated using the following equation:

$$\frac{\text{weight (kg)}}{\text{height (m)} \times \text{height (m)}}$$

So, a person weighing 56kg who is 1.5m tall has a BMI of 25:
$56 \div (1.5 \times 1.5) = 25$.
Alternatively:

$$\frac{\text{weight (lb)} \times 703}{\text{height (in)} \times \text{height (in)}}$$

So, the same person, weighing 123lb who is 59 in tall has the same BMI of 25:
$123 \times 703 \div (59 \times 59) = 25$.

BMI RATINGS

below 20:	underweight
20–24.9:	normal weight
25–29.9:	overweight
30–39.9:	moderate obesity
Over 40:	severe obesity

Balanced diets

Including foods from the five food groups means that you are meeting your requirements for nutrients.

THE FIVE GROUPS ARE:

1 Bread, cereals and potatoes. This group is rich in starchy carbohydrates and includes breakfast cereals, rice, pasta, noodles, yams and oats and should form the basis of most meals. Foods in this group are rich in insoluble fibre, calcium, iron and B vitamins, which are needed to keep your gut, bones and blood healthy. Try to eat wholegrain, wholemeal or high-fibre versions of breads and cereals.

2 Fruits and vegetables.

These are important sources of antioxidants such as vitamin C and beta-carotene (vegetable vitamin A), which protect us from cancers and heart disease. They are also rich in soluble fibre, which helps lower blood cholesterol. Try to include five portions of different fruits and vegetables in your diet each day, whether fresh, frozen, canned, dried or juiced.

A portion of fruit equals:
- 1 slice of pineapple, grapefruit, melon or watermelon, or half a mango or papaya
- 1 whole apple, avocado, banana, orange, peach or pear
- 2 small apricots, clementines, figs, kiwi fruit, passion fruit, plums, satsumas or tomatoes
- 1 cupful of berries, cherries or grapes
- 3 tablespoons stewed or canned apples, apricots, fruit cocktail, pears, peaches or pineapple, or fresh fruit salad
- 1 tablespoon dried apricots, bananas, cranberries, dates, figs, papaya, pineapple, raisins or sultanas
- 1 (150ml/5floz) glass of fruit juice (not fruit drinks or fruit squashes)

A portion of vegetables equals:
- 2 tablespoons broccoli, brussels sprouts, cabbage, cauliflower, radishes, turnip, swede, chard, winter greens, kale, pak choi, rocket, romaine lettuce, spinach, aubergine, carrots, green beans, mushrooms, onions, peas, peppers or squash
- half a cupful of alfalfa, baked beans, beansprouts, sprouting broccoli, black beans, chickpeas, kidney beans, lentils or soya beans
- 1 dessert bowl of salad
- 1 (150ml/5floz) glass of carrot, beetroot or wheatgrass juice

3 Milk and dairy foods.

These are excellent sources of calcium, protein and vitamins A and B12, essential for maintaining the health of bones, skin and blood. Include a couple of reduced-fat servings from this food group each day.

4 Meat, fish and alternatives.

The main nutrients supplied by this food group include iron, protein, B vitamins, zinc and magnesium, which help to maintain healthy blood and an efficient immune system. Choose at most two servings of lean red meat, fish, chicken, nuts, turkey, eggs, beans or pulses. The last two are great protein alternatives, as is tofu, which is also a good source of calcium.

5 Foods containing sugar or fat. Minimize your intake of savoury snacks, biscuits, cakes, crisps, pastries, sweets, chocolate, pies, butter and carbonated drinks, as these will hinder your efforts to lose weight.

Watch the fat

Gram for gram, fat has more than twice as many calories as protein and carbohydrates:

Calories per gram	kcal	kJ
fat	9	37
protein	4	17
carbohydrate	3.75	16

Foods with high levels of fat tend to be low in fibre and are not filling, so we eat more of these than high-carbohydrate foods. This raises the calorie intake even farther. Most of us should eat at least 25g (1oz) less fat a day.

GOOD FAT, BAD FAT
All fats will increase your weight if you eat too much, but not all raise the risk of developing disease. There are three types of fat: saturated, monounsaturated and polyunsaturated. The former raise levels of 'bad' cholesterol in the blood. Cholesterol is carried around

the body by two proteins: low-density lipoprotein (LDL) and high-density lipoprotein (HDL). When levels of LDL cholesterol are raised in the blood, it may be deposited on the blood vessel walls, narrowing them so they become blocked. If blood supply to the heart is interrupted it can lead to a heart attack which in severe cases can be fatal.

HDL is considered good as it carries cholesterol from various parts of the body to the liver where it can be disposed of.

As a general rule, fats that are hard at room temperature will contain the most saturated fat. Cakes, butter, cheese, biscuits, cooking fats, pastries, pies, fatty meat, whole milk and hard margarine provide the most saturated fats in our diets so cut down on these.

The monounsaturated and polyunsaturated fats are found in vegetable oils and fat spreads, and are considered healthier than saturated fats. Replacing the latter with the other versions can lower levels of LDL cholesterol.

Fatty or oily fish like sardines, salmon, mackerel, herring and trout contain polyunsaturated fats called omega-3 fats. These help to protect against heart disease. We should eat a serving of oily fish each week.

Guideline Daily Amounts

Guideline Daily Amounts (GDAs) are daily guideline figures recommended by health professionals for intake of calories, fat and saturates for adult women and men. These are average figures and personal requirements will vary with age, weight and levels of activity.

AVERAGE DAILY REQUIREMENT

	women	men
kcal	2000	2500
fat	70g	95g
saturates	20g	30g

Dietary Reference Values

Dietary Reference Values (DRVs) are daily recommendations set by the Department of Health for the nutrients considered sufficient for most adults and children in the UK. The table below gives the average daily requirement for protein, carbohydrate and fibre. If you are trying to lose weight, you will need less, and should discuss the exact amounts with your doctor or dietician.

AVERAGE DAILY REQUIREMENT

	women	men
protein	46g	56g
carbohydrate	225g	300g
fibre	18g	18g

How to use this book

It lists the energy, as kilocalories (kcal) and kilojoules (kJ), fat, saturated fat, protein, carbohydrate and fibre contained in more than 1500 foods. Nutrient values have been expressed as average servings so no calculator is needed.

The information shows where the energy comes from in any food so, if you're on a low-fat, low-carbohydrate diet or have any other special requirements, you can work out exactly how much you can have of any food.

Note

The average portion sizes of foods were obtained from *Food Portion Sizes, Second Edition,* HMSO, 1999. This information is based on a) weighed dietary surveys conducted by the Ministry of Agriculture, Fisheries and Food, b) information from manufacturers and c) by weighing numerous samples of foods such as takeaway dishes.

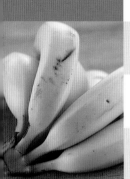

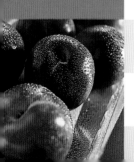

FRUITS	AVERAGE PORTION g
Apples, cooking	130
Apples, cooking, stewed with sugar	110
Apples, cooking, stewed without sugar	85
Apples, Cox's Pippin	100
Apples, Golden Delicious	100
Apples, Granny Smith	100
Apples, red dessert	100
Apricots	80
Apricots, canned in juice	140
Apricots, dried	120
Apricots, stewed with sugar	140
Apricots, stewed without sugar	140
Avocado, Fuerte	173
Avocado, Hass	173
Banana chips	13
Bananas	100
Bilberries	40
Blackberries	100
Blackberries, stewed with sugar	140
Blackberries, stewed without sugar	140
Blackcurrants	100
Blackcurrants, canned in juice	140
Blackcurrants, canned in syrup	140
Blackcurrants, stewed with sugar	140
Blackcurrants, stewed without sugar	140
Carambola	120
Cherries	80
Cherries, canned in syrup	68
Cherries, glacé	15
Clementines	60
Cranberries	75
Currants	25
Custard apples	60
Damsons	80

Unless otherwise stated, fruits are prepared but uncooked.

ENERGY kcal	ENERGY kJ	FAT g	SATURATED FAT g	PROTEIN g	CARBOHYDRATE g	FIBRE g
46	196	Trace	Trace	0	12	2.1
81	345	Trace	Trace	0	21	1.3
28	117	Trace	Trace	0	7	1.3
46	195	Trace	Trace	1	11	2
43	185	Trace	Trace	0	11	1.7
45	193	Trace	Trace	0	12	1.7
51	217	Trace	Trace	0	13	1.9
25	107	Trace	Trace	1	6	1.4
48	206	Trace	Trace	1	12	1.3
190	809	1	Trace	5	44	7.6
101	431	Trace	Trace	1	26	2.2
38	161	Trace	Trace	1	9	2.1
327	1349	33	6.1	4	3	5.9
330	1362	34	8.1	3	3	5.9
66	278	4	Trace	0	8	0.2
95	403	1	0.1	1	23	1.1
12	51	Trace	Trace	0	3	0.7
25	104	Trace	Trace	1	5	3.1
78	335	Trace	Trace	1	19	3.4
29	123	Trace	Trace	1	6	3.6
28	121	Trace	Trace	1	7	3.6
43	189	Trace	Trace	1	11	4.3
101	428	Trace	Trace	1	26	3.6
81	353	Trace	Trace	1	21	3.9
34	144	Trace	Trace	1	8	4.3
38	163	1	0.1	1	9	1.6
38	162	Trace	Trace	1	9	0.7
48	207	Trace	Trace	0	13	0.4
39	159	Trace	Trace	0	9	0
22	95	Trace	Trace	1	5	0.7
11	49	Trace	Trace	0	3	2.3
67	285	Trace	Trace	1	17	0.5
41	178	Trace	Trace	1	10	1.4
30	130	Trace	Trace	0	8	1.4

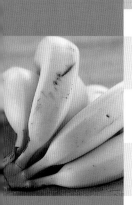

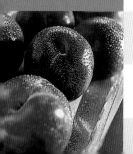

FRUITS	AVERAGE PORTION g
Damsons, stewed with sugar	100
Damsons, stewed without sugar	100
Dates	100
Dates, stoned and dried	60
Durian	80
Figs	55
Figs, dried	84
Fruit cocktail, canned in juice	115
Fruit cocktail, canned in syrup	115
Fruit salad, mixed	140
Gooseberries	100
Gooseberries, canned in syrup	140
Gooseberries, stewed with sugar	140
Gooseberries, stewed without sugar	140
Grapefruit	231
Grapefruit, canned in juice	120
Grapefruit, canned in syrup	120
Grapes	100
Greengages	100
Greengages, stewed with sugar	100
Greengages, stewed without sugar	100
Guavas	100
Guavas, canned in syrup	113
Kiwi fruit	60
Kumquats	8
Kumquats, canned in syrup	8
Lemons, unpeeled	60
Limes, unpeeled	40
Loganberries, canned in juice	140
Loganberries, stewed with sugar	140
Loganberries, stewed without sugar	140
Lychees	90
Lychees, canned in syrup	80
Mandarin oranges, canned in juice	115

Unless otherwise stated, fruits are prepared but uncooked.

ENERGY kcal	ENERGY kJ	FAT g	SATURATED FAT g	PROTEIN g	CARBOHYDRATE g	FIBRE g
74	316	Trace	Trace	0	19	1.5
34	147	Trace	Trace	1	9	1.6
124	530	Trace	Trace	2	31	1.8
162	691	1	0.1	2	41	2.4
109	460	1	Trace	2	23	3
24	102	1	0.1	1	5	0.8
176	747	1	Trace	3	41	5.8
33	140	Trace	Trace	0	8	1.2
66	281	Trace	Trace	0	17	1.2
77	332	Trace	Trace	1	19	2.1
40	170	1	0.1	1	9	2.4
102	434	Trace	Trace	1	26	2.4
76	321	Trace	Trace	1	18	2.7
22	92	Trace	Trace	1	4	2.8
69	291	Trace	Trace	2	16	3
36	144	Trace	Trace	1	9	0.5
72	308	Trace	Trace	1	19	0.7
60	257	Trace	Trace	0	15	0.7
41	173	Trace	Trace	1	10	2.1
81	347	Trace	Trace	1	21	1.9
36	155	Trace	Trace	1	9	1.9
26	112	1	Trace	1	5	3.7
68	292	Trace	Trace	0	18	3.4
29	124	Trace	Trace	1	6	1.1
3	15	Trace	Trace	0	1	0.3
11	46	Trace	Trace	0	3	0.1
8	36	1	0.1	0	1	1.7
4	14	0	0	0	0	1.1
141	601	Trace	Trace	1	37	2.2
70	300	Trace	Trace	1	18	2.8
20	87	Trace	Trace	1	4	2.9
52	223	Trace	Trace	1	13	0.6
54	232	Trace	Trace	0	14	0.4
37	155	Trace	Trace	1	9	0.3

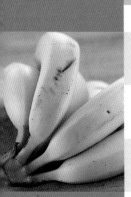

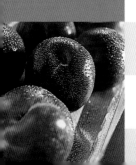

FRUITS	AVERAGE PORTION g
Mandarin oranges, canned in syrup	126
Mangoes	150
Mangoes, canned in syrup	105
Mangosteen	60
Melon, Canteloupe	150
Melon, Galia	150
Melon, Honeydew	200
Mixed peel	5
Nectarines	150
Oranges	160
Papaya	140
Passion fruit	60
Peaches	110
Peaches, canned in juice	120
Peaches, canned in syrup	120
Pears, canned in juice	135
Pears, canned in syrup	135
Pears, Comice	150
Pears, Conference	170
Pears, Nashi	150
Pears, William	150
Physalis	60
Pineapple	80
Pineapple, canned in juice	40
Pineapple, canned in syrup	40
Plums, average, stewed with sugar	133
Plums, average, stewed without sugar	70
Plums, canned in syrup	80
Plums, Victoria	55
Plums, yellow	55
Pomegranate	55
Pomelo	80
Prickly pears	60
Prunes, canned in juice	24

Unless otherwise stated, fruits are prepared but uncooked.

ENERGY kcal	ENERGY kJ	FAT g	SATURATED FAT g	PROTEIN g	CARBOHYDRATE g	FIBRE g
66	281	Trace	Trace	1	17	0.3
86	368	1	0.2	1	21	3.9
81	347	Trace	Trace	0	21	0.7
44	184	Trace	Trace	0	10	1
29	122	Trace	Trace	1	6	1.5
36	153	Trace	Trace	1	8	0.6
56	238	Trace	Trace	1	13	1.2
12	49	Trace	Trace	0	3	0.2
60	257	Trace	Trace	2	14	1.8
59	253	Trace	Trace	2	14	2.7
50	214	Trace	Trace	1	12	3.1
22	91	1	0.1	2	3	2
36	156	Trace	Trace	1	8	1.7
47	198	Trace	Trace	1	12	1
66	280	Trace	Trace	1	17	1.1
45	190	Trace	Trace	0	11	1.9
68	290	Trace	Trace	0	18	1.5
50	212	Trace	Trace	0	13	3
90	386	1	Trace	1	22	4.1
44	183	Trace	Trace	0	11	2.3
51	215	Trace	Trace	1	12	3.3
32	131	Trace	Trace	1	7	1
33	141	Trace	Trace	0	8	1
19	80	Trace	Trace	0	5	0.2
26	109	Trace	Trace	0	7	0.3
105	446	Trace	Trace	1	27	1.7
21	90	Trace	Trace	0	5	0.9
47	202	Trace	Trace	0	12	0.6
21	92	Trace	Trace	0	5	1
14	59	Trace	Trace	0	3	0.6
28	120	Trace	Trace	1	6	1.9
24	101	Trace	Trace	0	5	0.8
29	124	1	0.1	0	7	2.2
19	80	Trace	Trace	0	5	0.6

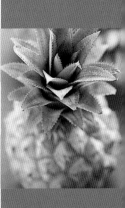

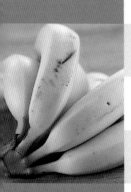

FRUITS	AVERAGE PORTION g
Prunes, canned in syrup	24
Prunes, dried	66
Prunes, stewed with sugar	24
Prunes, stewed without sugar	24
Quinces	90
Raisins	30
Rambutan	80
Raspberries	60
Raspberries, canned in syrup	90
Raspberries, stewed with sugar	90
Raspberries, stewed without sugar	90
Redcurrants	2
Redcurrants, stewed with sugar	140
Redcurrants, stewed without sugar	140
Rhubarb, canned in syrup	140
Rhubarb, stewed with sugar	140
Rhubarb, stewed without sugar	140
Satsumas	70
Sharon fruit	110
Starfruit	120
Strawberries	100
Sugar apples	60
Sultanas	18
Tangerines	70
Watermelon	200

Unless otherwise stated, fruits are prepared but uncooked.

ENERGY kcal	ENERGY kJ	FAT g	SATURATED FAT g	PROTEIN g	CARBOHYDRATE g	FIBRE g
22	93	Trace	Trace	0	6	0.7
93	397	Trace	Trace	2	22	3.8
25	105	Trace	Trace	0	6	0.7
19	83	Trace	0	0	5	0.8
23	99	Trace	Trace	0	6	1.7
82	348	Trace	Trace	1	21	0.6
55	234	Trace	Trace	1	13	0.5
15	65	1	0.1	1	3	1.5
79	337	Trace	Trace	1	20	1.4
57	244	1	0.1	1	14	2
22	95	1	0.1	1	4	2.2
0	2	Trace	Trace	0	0	0.1
74	318	Trace	Trace	1	19	3.8
24	106	Trace	Trace	1	5	4.1
43	182	Trace	Trace	1	11	1.1
67	284	Trace	Trace	1	16	1.7
10	42	Trace	Trace	1	1	1.8
25	109	Trace	Trace	1	6	0.9
80	342	Trace	Trace	1	20	1.8
38	163	1	0.1	1	9	1.6
27	113	Trace	Trace	1	6	1.1
41	178	Trace	Trace	1	10	1.4
50	211	Trace	Trace	0	12	0.4
25	103	Trace	Trace	1	6	0.9
62	266	1	0.2	1	14	0.2

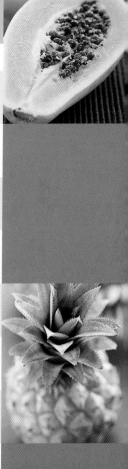

VEGETABLES	AVERAGE PORTION g
Ackee, canned	80
Alfalfa sprouts	5
Artichoke, globe, heart	40
Artichoke, Jerusalem	56
Asparagus	125
Aubergine, fried	130
Bamboo shoots, canned	50
Beans	
Aduki, dried, boiled	60
Baked, canned in tomato sauce	135
Baked, canned in tomato sauce, reduced sugar and salt	135
Baked, canned in tomato sauce, with burgers	225
Baked, canned in tomato sauce, with pork sausages	225
Balor, canned	135
Barbecue, canned in sauce	135
Blackeye, dried, boiled	60
Broad	120
Broad, canned	120
Broad, frozen	120
Butter, canned	120
Butter, dried, boiled	60
Chickpeas, canned	70
Chickpeas, split, dried, boiled	70
Chickpeas, whole, dried, boiled	70
Chilli, canned	135
French	90
French, canned	90
French, frozen	90
Green	90
Green, canned	90
Green, frozen	90

Unless otherwise stated, vegetables are described as they would normally be eaten.

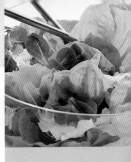

ENERGY kcal	ENERGY kJ	FAT g	SATURATED FAT g	PROTEIN g	CARBOHYDRATE g	FIBRE g
121	500	12	Trace	2	1	1.4
1	5	Trace	Trace	0	0	0.1
7	31	0	0	1	1	2
23	116	Trace	Trace	1	6	2
33	138	1	0.1	4	2	1.7
393	1620	41	5.3	2	4	3
6	23	1	0.1	1	0	0.9
74	315	Trace	Trace	6	14	3.3
109	466	1	0.1	6	20	4.7
99	420	1	0.1	7	17	5.1
214	900	7	0.1	15	25	6.8
239	1001	10	0.1	14	25	6.3
26	112	Trace	Trace	3	4	3.6
104	444	1	0.1	7	19	4.7
70	296	1	0.1	5	12	2.1
58	245	1	0.1	6	7	6.5
104	444	1	0.1	10	15	6.2
97	413	1	0.1	9	14	7.8
92	392	1	0.1	7	16	5.5
62	262	1	0.1	4	11	3.1
81	341	2	0.2	5	11	2.9
80	339	1	0.1	5	12	3
85	358	1	0.1	6	13	3
95	513	1	0.1	7	16	5.3
20	83	1	0.1	2	3	2.2
20	86	Trace	Trace	1	4	2.3
23	97	Trace	Trace	2	4	3.7
20	83	1	0.1	2	3	2.2
20	86	Trace	Trace	1	4	2.3
23	97	Trace	Trace	2	4	3.7

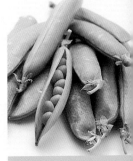

VEGETABLES
& SALADS **17**

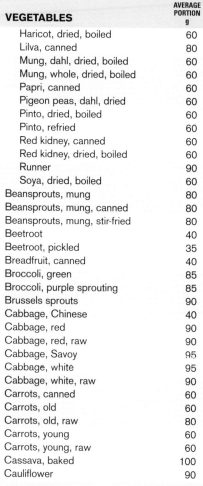

VEGETABLES	AVERAGE PORTION g
Haricot, dried, boiled	60
Lilva, canned	80
Mung, dahl, dried, boiled	60
Mung, whole, dried, boiled	60
Papri, canned	60
Pigeon peas, dahl, dried	60
Pinto, dried, boiled	60
Pinto, refried	60
Red kidney, canned	60
Red kidney, dried, boiled	60
Runner	90
Soya, dried, boiled	60
Beansprouts, mung	80
Beansprouts, mung, canned	80
Beansprouts, mung, stir-fried	80
Beetroot	40
Beetroot, pickled	35
Breadfruit, canned	40
Broccoli, green	85
Broccoli, purple sprouting	85
Brussels sprouts	90
Cabbage, Chinese	40
Cabbage, red	90
Cabbage, red, raw	90
Cabbage, Savoy	95
Cabbage, white	95
Cabbage, white, raw	90
Carrots, canned	60
Carrots, old	60
Carrots, old, raw	80
Carrots, young	60
Carrots, young, raw	60
Cassava, baked	100
Cauliflower	90

Unless otherwise stated, vegetables are described as they would normally be eaten.

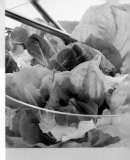

ENERGY kcal	ENERGY kJ	FAT g	SATURATED FAT g	PROTEIN g	CARBOHYDRATE g	FIBRE g
57	244	1	0.1	4	10	3.7
54	232	1	0.1	5	8	0.5
55	235	1	0.1	5	9	1.8
55	233	1	0.1	5	9	1.8
16	66	1	0.1	2	2	0.4
71	298	1	0.1	5	13	4
82	350	1	0.1	5	14	2.8
64	268	1	0.1	4	9	3.2
60	254	1	0.1	4	11	3.7
62	264	1	0.1	5	10	4
16	68	1	0.1	1	2	1.7
85	354	4	0.5	8	3	3.7
25	105	1	0.1	2	3	1.2
8	35	Trace	Trace	1	1	0.6
58	238	5	0.4	2	2	0.7
18	78	Trace	Trace	1	4	0.8
10	41	Trace	Trace	0	2	0.6
26	112	Trace	Trace	0	7	0.7
20	85	1	0.2	3	1	2
16	68	1	0.1	2	1	2
32	138	1	0.3	3	3	2.8
5	20	Trace	Trace	0	1	0.5
14	55	Trace	Trace	1	2	1.8
19	80	Trace	Trace	1	3	2.3
16	67	1	0.1	1	2	1.9
13	57	Trace	Trace	1	2	1.4
24	102	Trace	Trace	1	5	1.9
12	52	1	0.1	0	3	1.1
14	60	1	0.1	0	3	1.5
28	117	1	0.1	0	6	1.9
13	56	1	0.1	0	3	1.4
18	75	1	0.1	0	4	1.4
155	661	1	0.1	1	40	1.7
25	105	1	0.2	3	2	1.4

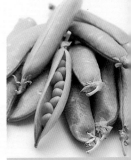

VEGETABLES
& SALADS

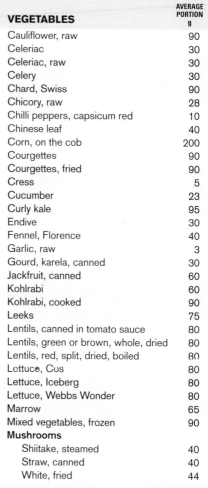

VEGETABLES	AVERAGE PORTION g
Cauliflower, raw	90
Celeriac	30
Celeriac, raw	30
Celery	30
Chard, Swiss	90
Chicory, raw	28
Chilli peppers, capsicum red	10
Chinese leaf	40
Corn, on the cob	200
Courgettes	90
Courgettes, fried	90
Cress	5
Cucumber	23
Curly kale	95
Endive	30
Fennel, Florence	40
Garlic, raw	3
Gourd, karela, canned	30
Jackfruit, canned	60
Kohlrabi	60
Kohlrabi, cooked	90
Leeks	75
Lentils, canned in tomato sauce	80
Lentils, green or brown, whole, dried	80
Lentils, red, split, dried, boiled	80
Lettuce, Cos	80
Lettuce, Iceberg	80
Lettuce, Webbs Wonder	80
Marrow	65
Mixed vegetables, frozen	90
Mushrooms	
Shiitake, steamed	40
Straw, canned	40
White, fried	44

Unless otherwise stated, vegetables are described as they would normally
be eaten.

ENERGY kcal	ENERGY kJ	FAT g	SATURATED FAT g	PROTEIN g	CARBOHYDRATE g	FIBRE g
31	128	1	0.2	3	3	1.6
5	19	Trace	Trace	0	1	1
5	22	Trace	Trace	0	1	1.1
2	10	Trace	Trace	0	0	0.3
18	76	Trace	Trace	2	3	1.8
3	13	1	0.1	0	1	0.3
3	11	Trace	Trace	0	0	0.1
5	20	Trace	Trace	0	1	0.5
132	560	3	0.4	5	23	2.6
17	73	1	0.1	2	2	1.1
57	239	4	0.5	2	2	1.1
1	3	Trace	Trace	0	0	0.1
2	9	Trace	Trace	0	0	0.1
23	95	1	0.2	2	1	2.7
4	16	0	0	1	0	0.6
5	20	Trace	Trace	0	1	1
3	12	0	0	0	0	0.1
3	11	Trace	Trace	0	0	0.7
62	264	Trace	Trace	0	16	0.9
14	57	Trace	Trace	1	2	1.3
16	69	Trace	Trace	1	3	1.7
16	65	1	0.1	1	2	1.3
44	189	Trace	Trace	4	7	1.4
84	357	1	0.1	7	14	3
80	339	Trace	Trace	6	14	1.5
13	52	1	0.1	1	1	1
10	42	Trace	Trace	1	2	0.5
10	44	Trace	Trace	1	2	0.6
6	25	Trace	Trace	0	1	0.4
38	162	Trace	Trace	3	6	2.9
22	93	Trace	0	1	5	0.8
6	25	Trace	Trace	1	0	1
69	284	7	0.9	1	0	0.7

VEGETABLES	AVERAGE PORTION g
White, raw	40
Okra	30
Onions	150
Onions, fried	40
Parsnips	65
Parsnips, roasted without oil	90
Peas, canned	70
Peas, fresh	70
Peas, frozen	70
Peas, mangetout, stir-fried	90
Peas, marrowfat, canned	80
Peas, mushy, canned	80
Peas, petit pois, canned	70
Peas, petit pois, frozen	70
Peas, sugar-snap	90
Pease pudding, canned	80
Peppers, capsicum, green	160
Peppers, capsicum, red	160
Peppers, capsicum, yellow	160
Plantain	200
Plantain, ripe, fried	200
Potatoes and potato products	
Chips, crinkle cut, frozen, fried	165
Chips, fine cut, frozen, fried	165
Chips, fried	165
Chips, shop bought, fried	165
Chips, straight cut, frozen, fried	165
Chips, thick cut, frozen, fried	165
Croquettes, fried	180
Duchesse	120
French fries	110
Microwave chips	165
Instant mash, made with semi-skimmed milk	60

Unless otherwise stated, vegetables are described as they would normally be eaten.

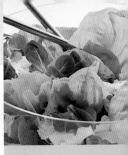

ENERGY kcal	ENERGY kJ	FAT g	SATURATED FAT g	PROTEIN g	CARBOHYDRATE g	FIBRE g
5	22	Trace	0	1	0	0.4
8	36	1	0.1	1	1	1.1
54	225	Trace	Trace	2	12	2.1
66	274	4	0.6	1	6	1.2
43	181	1	0.1	1	8	3.1
102	427	6	Trace	1	12	4.2
56	237	1	0.1	4	9	3.6
55	230	1	0.2	5	7	3.2
48	204	1	0.1	4	7	3.6
64	268	4	0.4	3	3	2.2
80	329	1	0.1	6	14	3.3
65	276	1	0.1	5	11	1.4
32	132	1	0.1	4	3	3
34	144	1	0.1	4	4	3.2
30	125	1	0.1	3	4	1.2
74	316	1	0.1	5	13	1.4
24	104	1	0.2	1	4	2.6
51	214	1	0.2	2	10	2.6
42	181	Trace	Trace	2	8	2.7
224	954	1	0.2	2	57	2.4
534	2252	1	2	3	95	4.6
479	2001	28	5.1	6	55	3.6
601	2515	35	6.6	7	68	4.5
312	1313	11	1.5	6	50	3.6
394	1652	20	2.6	5	50	3.6
450	1889	22	4.1	7	59	4
386	1622	17	3.1	6	56	4
385	1607	24	3.1	7	39	2.3
148	622	6	3.6	4	20	1.4
308	1291	17	6.4	4	37	2.3
365	1535	17	3	6	53	4.8
42	178	1	0.2	1	9	0.6

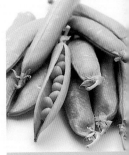

VEGETABLES
& SALADS 23

VEGETABLES

	AVERAGE PORTION g
Instant mash, made with water	60
Instant mash, made with whole milk	60
New, canned	165
New, chipped, fried	165
New, in skins, boiled	175
Old, baked	180
Old, boiled	175
Old, mashed with butter	120
Old, mashed with polyunsaturated fat spread	120
Old, roast	130
Oven chips, frozen	165
Oven chips, thick cut, frozen	165
Waffles, frozen	90
Wedges, baked	180
Pumpkin	60
Raddiccio, raw	30
Radishes, red, raw	48
Salad onions	10
Sauerkraut	30
Spinach	90
Spinach, cooked	90
Split peas, dried, boiled	90
Spring greens, boiled	95
Spring onions	10
Squash, acorn, baked	65
Squash, butternut, baked	65
Squash, spaghetti, baked	65
Swede	60
Sweet potato	130
Sweet potato, baked	130
Sweetcorn, baby, canned	60
Sweetcorn kernels, canned, reheated	85
Tomatoes	85

Unless otherwise stated, vegetables are described as they would normally be eaten.

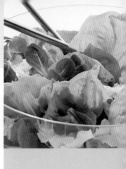

ENERGY kcal	ENERGY kJ	FAT g	SATURATED FAT g	PROTEIN g	CARBOHYDRATE g	FIBRE g
34	147	Trace	Trace	1	8	0.6
46	193	1	0.4	1	9	0.6
104	447	Trace	Trace	2	25	1.3
376	1582	16	2	7	55	2.8
116	492	1	0.2	2	27	2.6
245	1046	Trace	Trace	7	57	4.9
126	536	Trace	Trace	3	30	2.1
125	526	5	3.4	2	19	1.3
125	526	5	1.1	2	19	1.3
194	819	6	0.8	4	34	2.3
267	1134	7	3	5	49	3.3
259	1096	7	2.8	5	46	3
180	758	12	1	2	28	2
245	1046	Trace	Trace	7	57	4.9
8	34	1	0.1	0	1	0.7
4	17	Trace	Trace	0	1	0.5
6	24	0	0	0	1	0.4
2	10	0	0	0	0	0.2
3	11	Trace	Trace	0	0	0.7
23	93	1	0.1	3	1	1.9
17	71	1	0.1	2	1	1.9
113	484	1	0.2	7	20	2.4
19	78	1	0.1	2	2	2.5
2	10	0	0	0	0	0.2
36	152	Trace	Trace	1	8	2.1
21	89	Trace	Trace	1	5	0.9
15	62	Trace	0.1	0	3	1.4
7	28	Trace	Trace	0	1	0.4
109	465	1	0.1	1	27	3
150	634	1	0.3	2	36	4.3
14	58	Trace	Trace	2	1	0.9
104	441	1	0.2	2	23	1.2
14	62	1	0.1	1	3	0.9

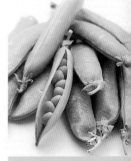

VEGETABLES
& SALADS

VEGETABLES

	AVERAGE PORTION g
Tomatoes, canned, not drained	200
Tomatoes, cherry	90
Tomatoes, fried	85
Tomatoes, grilled	85
Turnips	60
Water chestnuts, canned	28
Watercress	20
Yam	130
Yam, baked	130
Yam, steamed	130

PREPARED SALADS

Baby leaf salad	50
Bean salad	200
Beetroot salad	100
Carrot and nut salad with French dressing	95
Coleslaw, with mayonnaise	100
Coleslaw, with reduced-calorie dressing	100
Coleslaw, with vinaigrette	100
Florida salad	95
Greek salad	95
Green salad	95
Herb salad	50
Pasta salad	95
Pasta salad, wholemeal	95
Potato salad, with mayonnaise	85
Potato salad, with reduced-calorie mayonnaise	85
Rice salad	90
Rice salad, brown	95
Rocket salad	25
Tabbouleh	100

Unless otherwise stated, vegetables are described as they would normally be eaten.

ENERGY kcal	ENERGY kJ	FAT g	SATURATED FAT g	PROTEIN g	CARBOHYDRATE g	FIBRE g
32	138	Trace	Trace	2	6	1.4
16	68	1	0.1	1	3	0.9
77	320	7	0.9	1	4	1.1
42	179	1	0.3	2	8	2.5
7	31	1	Trace	0	1	1.1
9	37	Trace	Trace	0	3	2
4	19	1	0.1	1	0	0.3
173	738	1	0.1	2	43	1.8
199	846	1	0.1	3	49	2.2
148	634	1	0.1	2	37	1.7
9	40	Trace	Trace	Trace	2	0.7
294	1236	19	2	8	26	6
100	417	7	0.7	2	8	1.7
207	858	17	1.6	2	13	2.3
258	939	26	3.9	1	4	1.4
67	280	5	0.5	1	6	1.4
87	364	4	0.5	1	12	1.7
213	790	19	2.9	1	9	1
124	513	12	3.1	3	2	0.8
11	48	0	Trace	1	2	1
9	40	Trace	Trace	Trace	Trace	0.7
121	473	7	1	2	13	1.5
124	493	7	1	3	13	2.6
203	757	18	2.6	1	10	0.8
82	349	3	0.3	1	13	0.7
149	628	7	1	3	21	0.6
159	668	7	1	3	23	1
3	12	Trace	Trace	Trace	Trace	0.2
119	496	5	0.4	3	17	1

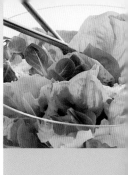

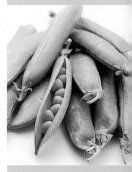

VEGETABLES
& SALADS **27**

PREPARED SALADS	AVERAGE PORTION g
Tomato and onion salad	90
Waldorf salad	90

VEGETABLE DISHES, HOMEMADE

Bean loaf	90
Bhaji, aubergine, pea, potato and cauliflower	70
Bhaji, potato and cauliflower, fried	70
Bhaji, potato and onion	70
Broccoli in cheese sauce, made with semi-skimmed milk	190
Broccoli in cheese sauce, made with whole milk	190
Bubble and squeak, fried	140
Cannelloni, spinach	340
Cannelloni, vegetable	340
Casserole, vegetable	220
Cauliflower cheese, made with semi-skimmed milk	200
Cauliflower cheese, made with whole milk	200
Cauliflower in white sauce, made with skimmed milk	200
Cauliflower in white sauce, made with whole milk	200
Chilli, bean and lentil	290
Chilli, vegetable	220
Curry, chickpea	210
Curry, potato and pea	290
Curry, vegetable	200
Dahl, mung bean, dried, boiled	60
Dahl, pigeon peas, dried, boiled	60
Falafel, fried	100

Unless otherwise stated, vegetables are described as they would normally be eaten.

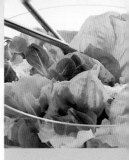

ENERGY kcal	ENERGY kJ	FAT g	SATURATED FAT g	PROTEIN g	CARBOHYDRATE g	FIBRE g
65	272	5	0.6	1	4	0.9
174	662	16	2.1	1	7	1.2
134	564	7	0.7	6	14	3.9
49	209	2	0.2	2	7	2
214	888	15	1.8	5	14	2.7
112	468	7	4.6	1	12	1.1
211	880	14	7.2	12	9	2.9
224	939	16	8.2	12	9	2.9
174	727	13	1.4	2	14	2.1
449	1880	26	7.8	15	43	2.7
493	2067	31	11.6	15	43	2.4
114	486	1	0.2	5	23	4.6
200	840	13	6	12	10	2.6
210	880	14	6.6	12	10	2.6
122	512	6	2.2	7	10	2.2
136	568	8	3.2	7	10	2.2
264	1111	8	0.9	15	38	10.4
125	532	1	0.2	7	24	5.7
227	956	8	0.8	13	30	6.9
267	1122	11	1.2	8	38	7
176	736	12	1.2	5	14	5
55	235	1	0.1	5	9	1.8
71	298	1	0.1	5	13	4
179	750	11	1.1	6	16	3.4

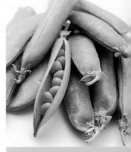

VEGETABLE DISHES, HOMEMADE	AVERAGE PORTION g
Lasagne, spinach	420
Lasagne, spinach, wholemeal	420
Lasagne, vegetable	420
Lasagne, vegetable, wholemeal	420
Lentil and nut roast	100
Lentil pie	100
Lentil roast	100
Moussaka, vegetable	330
Pakora, potato and cauliflower, fried	70
Pasty, vegetable	155
Pasty, vegetable, wholemeal	155
Peppers, stuffed with rice	175
Peppers, stuffed with vegetables, cheese topping	175
Pilau, mushroom	180
Pilau, vegetable	180
Quiche, broccoli	140
Quiche, broccoli, wholemeal	140
Quiche, cauliflower cheese	140
Quiche, cauliflower cheese, wholemeal	140
Quiche, cheese and egg	140
Quiche, cheese and egg, wholemeal	140
Quiche, cheese and mushroom	140
Quiche, cheese and mushroom, wholemeal	140
Quiche, cheese, onion and potato	140
Quiche, cheese, onion and potato, wholemeal	140
Quiche, mushroom	140
Quiche, mushroom, wholemeal	140
Quiche, spinach	140
Quiche, spinach, wholemeal	140
Quiche, vegetable	140
Quiche, vegetable, wholemeal	140

Unless otherwise stated, vegetables are described as they would normally be eaten.

ENERGY kcal	ENERGY kJ	FAT g	SATURATED FAT g	PROTEIN g	CARBOHYDRATE g	FIBRE g
365	1541	13	5.5	15	53	4.6
391	1659	13	5.5	18	55	9.7
428	1810	18	9.2	17	52	4.2
445	1877	19	9.2	20	52	8.8
222	929	12	1.8	11	19	3.8
156	659	4	0.5	7	24	3.8
139	588	3	0.4	8	22	3.4
452	1888	31	9.2	15	30	4
214	888	15	1.8	5	14	2.7
425	1783	23	5.7	6	52	2.9
406	1702	24	5.7	8	43	6.4
149	630	4	0.7	3	27	2.3
194	810	12	3.5	6	17	2.6
248	1048	8	4.5	4	43	0.7
248	1053	8	4.3	5	43	1
349	1455	21	8.3	12	30	1.7
337	1408	21	8.3	13	25	3.8
277	1156	18	7.1	7	24	1.5
269	1121	18	7.1	8	20	3.1
440	1834	31	14.4	18	24	0.8
431	1796	31	14.6	18	20	2.7
396	1655	26	10.8	15	26	1.3
388	1616	27	10.8	16	22	3.1
480	2005	33	16	18	28	1.4
472	1966	34	16.1	19	25	3.1
398	1659	27	12.2	14	26	1.3
388	1618	28	12.2	15	21	3.1
287	1203	18	5.6	14	18	2
281	1176	18	5.6	15	16	3.2
295	1238	18	6	7	28	2.1
286	1197	18	6	8	24	3.9

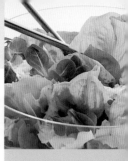

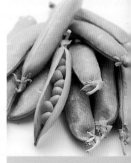

VEGETABLE DISHES, HOMEMADE

	AVERAGE PORTION g
Refried beans	90
Rice and blackeye beans	200
Rice and blackeye beans, brown rice	200
Risotto, vegetable	290
Risotto, vegetable, brown rice	290
Rissoles, chickpea, fried	100
Rissoles, lentil, fried	100
Vegetable bake	260
Vine leaves, stuffed with rice	80

VEGETARIAN PRODUCTS AND DISHES

Beanburger, aduki, fried	90
Beanburger, butter bean, fried	90
Beanburger, red kidney bean, fried	90
Beanburger, soya, fried	90
Quorn™, myco-protein	90
Tempeh	60
Tofu, fried	80
Tofu, steamed	80
Tofu, steamed, fried	80
Tofu burger, baked	9
Vegebanger mix, made with water and egg, fried	56
Vegebanger mix, made with water, fried	56
Vegeburger, fried	56
Vegeburger, grilled	56
Vegeburger mix, made with water and egg, fried	56
Vegeburger mix, made with water and egg, grilled	56
Vegeburger mix, made with water, fried	56
Vegeburger mix, made with water, grilled	56

Unless otherwise stated, vegetables are described as they would normally be eaten.

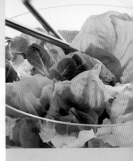

ENERGY kcal	ENERGY kJ	FAT g	SATURATED FAT g	PROTEIN g	CARBOHYDRATE g	FIBRE g
211	885	12	2.7	9	18	6.3
366	1556	7	3	12	68	2.8
350	1488	7	3	11	66	3.6
426	1798	19	2.9	12	56	6.4
415	1749	19	2.6	12	54	7
243	1016	17	1.9	8	16	4.1
211	886	11	1.3	9	22	3.6
330	1383	18	7.8	11	32	2.9
210	875	14	2.1	2	19	1.0
165	695	6	0.9	7	21	3.9
172	722	10	1.1	5	17	3.7
183	768	10	1.1	6	20	4.4
174	725	10	1.4	10	12	4.2
77	326	3	Trace	11	2	4.3
100	418	4	2	12	4	2.6
242	1011	20	2.3	17	3	1
58	243	3	0.4	6	1	1
209	869	14	2.3	19	2	1
11	45	0	0.1	1	1	0.2
157	659	10	2.5	10	7	1.9
137	572	9	2	8	7	1.8
137	571	10	1.7	9	4	2
110	460	6	1.7	9	4	2.4
122	511	7	1.6	8	7	1.8
91	385	4	1.2	8	7	1.8
115	482	6	1.3	7	8	2
84	356	3	1	7	8	2

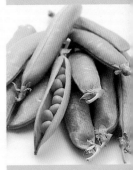

VEGETABLES
& SALADS **33**

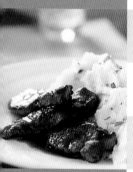

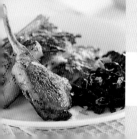

BEEF	AVERAGE PORTION g
Braising steak, braised	140
Braising steak, untrimmed, braised	140
Braising steak, slow cooked	140
Braising steak, untrimmed, slow cooked	140
Fillet steak, fried	172
Fillet steak, untrimmed, fried	172
Fillet steak, grilled	168
Fillet steak, untrimmed, grilled	168
Flank, pot roasted	140
Flank, untrimmed, pot roasted	140
Fore rib, roasted	90
Fore rib, untrimmed, roasted	90
Mince, extra lean, stewed	140
Mince, microwaved	140
Mince, stewed	140
Rib roast, roasted	90
Rib roast, untrimmed, roasted	90
Rump steak, grilled	163
Rump steak, untrimmed, grilled	163
Rump steak, fried	166
Rump steak, untrimmed, fried	166
Rump steak strips, stir-fried	103
Rump steak strips, untrimmed, stir-fried	103
Silverside, pot roasted	140
Silverside, untrimmed, pot roasted	140
Silverside, salted, boiled	140
Silverside, untrimmed, salted, boiled	140
Sirloin joint, roasted	90
Sirloin joint, untrimmed, roasted	90
Sirloin steak, fried	169
Sirloin steak, untrimmed, fried	169
Sirloin steak, grilled medium rare	166
Sirloin steak, untrimmed, grilled medium rare	166

Unless otherwise stated, all meat is lean and trimmed, and all chops and
cutlets are boned. Steaks are medium-sized. Unless stated otherwise, all
dishes are homemade.

ENERGY kcal	ENERGY kJ	FAT g	SATURATED FAT g	PROTEIN g	CARBOHYDRATE g	FIBRE g
315	1322	14	5.7	48	0	0
344	1441	18	7.4	46	0	0
276	1156	11	4.8	44	0	0
304	1270	16	6.7	41	0	0
316	1328	14	5.8	49	0	0
330	1384	15	6.7	49	0	0
316	1329	13	6	49	0	0
336	1410	16	7.4	48	0	0
354	1483	20	8	45	0	0
433	1800	31	12.7	38	0	0
212	889	10	4.6	30	0	0
270	1125	18	8.3	26	0	0
248	1039	12	5.3	35	0	0
368	1534	25	10.6	37	0	0
293	1218	19	8.3	31	0	0
212	889	10	4.6	30	0	0
270	1125	18	8.3	26	0	0
287	1208	9	3.9	51	0	0
331	1384	15	6.5	48	0	0
304	1278	11	4.2	51	0	0
378	1582	21	8.1	47	0	0
214	901	9	3.4	33	0	0
255	1069	15	5.8	31	0	0
270	1135	9	3.5	48	0	0
346	1448	19	7.8	43	0	0
258	1081	10	3.5	43	0	0
314	1312	18	6.6	39	0	0
169	712	6	2.6	29	0	0
210	876	11	5	27	0	0
319	1340	14	5.7	49	0	0
394	1646	24	10.1	45	0	0
292	1223	13	5.6	44	0	0
354	1474	21	9.3	41	0	0

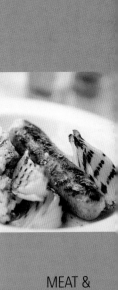

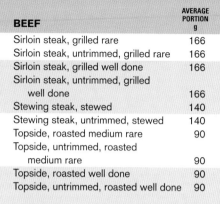

BEEF

	AVERAGE PORTION g
Sirloin steak, grilled rare	166
Sirloin steak, untrimmed, grilled rare	166
Sirloin steak, grilled well done	166
Sirloin steak, untrimmed, grilled well done	166
Stewing steak, stewed	140
Stewing steak, untrimmed, stewed	140
Topside, roasted medium rare	90
Topside, untrimmed, roasted medium rare	90
Topside, roasted well done	90
Topside, untrimmed, roasted well done	90

LAMB

Best end neck cutlets, grilled	50
Best end neck cutlets, untrimmed, grilled	50
Breast, roasted	90
Breast, untrimmed, roasted	90
Chump chops, fried	70
Chump chops, untrimmed, fried	70
Chump steaks, untrimmed, fried	90
Kebabs, grilled	90
Leg, roasted medium	90
Leg, untrimmed, roasted medium	90
Leg, roasted well done	90
Leg, untrimmed, roasted well done	90
Leg chops, untrimmed, grilled	70
Leg half fillet, braised	70
Leg half fillet, untrimmed, braised	70
Leg half knuckle, pot roasted	90
Leg half knuckle, untrimmed, pot roasted	90
Leg joint, roasted	90

Unless otherwise stated, all meat is lean and trimmed, and all chops and
cutlets are boned. Steaks are medium-sized. Unless stated otherwise, all
dishes are homemade.

ENERGY kcal	ENERGY kJ	FAT g	SATURATED FAT g	PROTEIN g	CARBOHYDRATE g	FIBRE g
276	1157	11	5	44	0	0
359	1494	21	9.6	42	0	0
374	1565	16	7.3	56	0	0
427	1781	24	10.8	53	0	0
259	1088	9	3.2	45	0	0
284	1193	13	5.2	41	0	0
158	662	5	1.9	29	0	0
200	837	10	4.3	27	0	0
182	764	6	2.3	33	0	0
220	918	11	4.7	30	0	0
118	493	7	3.3	14	0	0
171	710	14	6.6	12	0	0
246	1024	17	7.7	24	0	0
323	1338	27	12.9	20	0	0
149	624	8	3.5	20	0	0
216	895	16	7.6	17	0	0
255	1058	18	8.5	22	0	0
259	1079	17	8.1	26	0	0
183	768	8	3.4	27	0	0
216	904	13	5.3	25	0	0
187	786	8	3.3	28	0	0
218	909	12	5.1	27	0	0
155	648	8	3.5	20	0	0
143	597	7	3.2	19	0	0
179	748	12	5.4	18	0	0
181	760	8	3.5	26	0	0
213	889	12	5.4	25	0	0
189	791	9	3.1	28	0	0

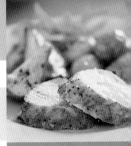

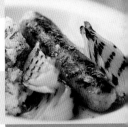

MEAT &
MEAT DISHES

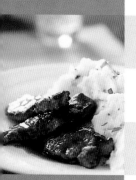

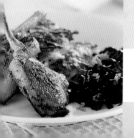

LAMB	AVERAGE PORTION g
Leg joint, untrimmed, roasted	90
Leg steaks, grilled	90
Leg steaks, untrimmed, grilled	90
Loin chops, grilled	70
Loin chops, untrimmed, grilled	70
Loin chops, roasted	70
Loin chops, untrimmed, roasted	70
Loin joint, roasted	90
Loin joint, untrimmed, roasted	90
Mince, stewed	90
Neck fillet, grilled	90
Neck fillet, untrimmed, grilled	90
Neck fillet strips, stir-fried	90
Neck fillet strips, untrimmed, stir-fried	90
Rack of lamb, roasted	90
Rack of lamb, untrimmed, roasted	90
Shoulder half bladeside, pot roasted	90
Shoulder half bladeside, untrimmed, pot roasted	90
Shoulder half knuckle, braised	90
Shoulder half knuckle, untrimmed, braised	90
Shoulder joint, roasted	90
Shoulder joint, untrimmed, roasted	90
Shoulder, roasted	90
Shoulder, untrimmed, roasted	90
Stewing lamb, stewed	260
Stewing lamb, untrimmed, stewed	260

Unless otherwise stated, all meat is lean and trimmed, and all chops and
cutlets are boned. Steaks are medium-sized. Unless stated otherwise, all
dishes are homemade.

ENERGY kcal	ENERGY kJ	FAT g	SATURATED FAT g	PROTEIN g	CARBOHYDRATE g	FIBRE g
212	887	12	4.2	27	0	0
178	746	8	3.2	26	0	0
208	868	12	5	25	0	0
149	624	7	3.4	20	0	0
214	888	15	7.4	19	0	0
180	754	9	4.3	24	0	0
251	1043	19	9	20	0	0
188	788	10	4.4	25	0	0
273	1133	20	9.5	23	0	0
187	783	11	5.2	22	0	0
256	1063	17	7.8	25	0	0
272	1131	20	9.3	24	0	0
250	1040	18	7.4	22	0	0
271	1124	21	8.9	21	0	0
203	848	12	5.6	24	0	0
327	1355	27	13.3	21	0	0
211	878	13	5.8	24	0	0
292	1212	23	10.8	21	0	0
191	797	11	4.9	23	0	0
272	1130	21	9.7	21	0	0
212	884	12	5.6	26	0	0
254	1056	18	8.4	23	0	0
196	819	11	5	24	0	0
268	1114	20	9.4	22	0	0
624	2600	38	16.9	69	0	0
725	3013	52	23.9	63	0	0

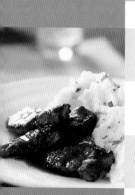

MEAT DISHES	AVERAGE PORTION g
Beef bourguignon	260
Beef casserole, canned	270
Beef casserole, made with canned cook-in sauce	300
Beef hotpot with potatoes, shop bought	260
Beef stew	280
Beef stew, made with lean beef	260
Beef stew and dumplings	260
Cannelloni, shop bought	260
Chilli con carne	220
Chilli con carne, shop bought	220
Corned beef hash	300
Cottage pie	310
Cottage pie, shop bought	310
Irish stew	330
Irish stew, made with lean beef	330
Lamb hotpot with potatoes, shop bought	260
Lancashire hotpot	260
Lasagne, shop bought	420
Meatloaf	100
Moussaka	330
Moussaka, shop bought	330
Pork and beef meatballs in tomato sauce	160
Pork casserole, made with canned cook-in sauce	260
Sausage casserole	350
Shepherd's pie	310
Shepherd's pie, shop bought	310
Toad in the hole	160
Toad in the hole, made with skimmed milk and reduced-fat sausages	160

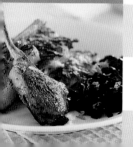

Unless otherwise stated, all meat is lean and trimmed, and all chops and cutlets are boned. Steaks are medium-sized. Unless stated otherwise, all dishes are homemade.

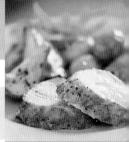

ENERGY kcal	ENERGY kJ	FAT g	SATURATED FAT g	PROTEIN g	CARBOHYDRATE g	FIBRE g
328	1368	17	5.5	36	7	1
211	886	7	3.8	19	19	2.7
408	1707	20	8.1	45	14	2.7
281	1183	11	4.4	19	28	2.3
316	1328	14	4.2	34	14	2
263	1102	9	2.3	32	13	1.8
499	2090	27	12.5	26	41	2.6
315	1326	13	5.2	17	35	3.1
286	1199	17	6.6	20	10	2.4
211	889	9	4.2	17	16	3.1
423	1776	18	9.9	31	37	3
391	1634	21	7.8	20	32	2.8
344	1448	17	7.4	14	37	2.8
399	1676	21	9.6	25	29	3.3
366	1541	17	7.3	26	29	3.3
281	1183	11	4.4	19	28	2.3
289	1206	14	5.5	23	20	2.3
601	2533	26	11.8	31	66	2.9
214	894	11	4.1	17	13	0.5
403	1680	26	11.9	28	15	3.3
462	1934	27	9.6	27	28	2.6
202	840	12	4.4	16	8	1.2
398	1664	20	6.8	44	10	0
578	2405	38	12.3	42	18	3.1
391	1634	21	7.8	20	32	2.8
344	1448	17	7.4	14	37	2.8
443	1853	28	10.7	19	31	1.8
320	1344	14	4.6	20	31	1.9

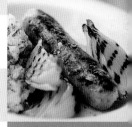

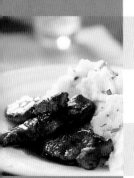

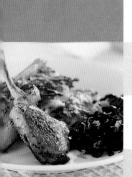

MEAT PRODUCTS	AVERAGE PORTION g
Black pudding, dry-fried	75
Corned beef	50
Faggots in gravy, shop bought	150
Haggis, boiled	85
Luncheon meat, canned	40
Meatloaf, shop bought	100
Scotch eggs, shop bought	120
White pudding	75

SAUSAGES	
Beef sausages, fried	40
Beef sausages, grilled	40
Bratwurst	75
Chorizo	30
Frankfurter	47
Garlic sausage	40
Kabana	30
Mortadella	24
Pastrami	50
Pork and beef sausages, grilled	40
Pork and beef, economy sausages, fried	40
Pork and beef, economy sausages, grilled	40
Pork sausages, fried	40
Pork sausages, grilled	40
Pork sausages, frozen, fried	40
Pork sausages, frozen, grilled	40
Pork sausages, reduced-fat, fried	40
Pork sausages, reduced-fat, grilled	40
Premium sausages, fried	40
Premium sausages, grilled	40
Salami	12
Saveloy, unbattered, shop bought	65

Unless otherwise stated, all meat is lean and trimmed, and all chops and
cutlets are boned. Steaks are medium-sized. Unless stated otherwise, all
dishes are homemade.

ENERGY kcal	ENERGY kJ	FAT g	SATURATED FAT g	PROTEIN g	CARBOHYDRATE g	FIBRE g
223	927	16	6.4	8	12	0.2
103	430	5	2.8	13	1	0
222	929	11	3.8	12	19	0.3
264	1098	18	6.5	9	16	0.2
112	463	10	3.5	5	1	0.1
216	900	16	5.6	17	1	0.5
301	1255	5.2	19	14	16	0
338	1407	24	8	5	27	1
112	464	8	3	5	5	0.3
111	463	8	3.2	5	5	0.3
195	811	16	6	12	2	Trace
87	362	7	2.9	5	1	Trace
135	559	12	4.3	6	1	0
99	412	8	2.9	6	0	Trace
92	383	8	3.4	5	0	Trace
79	328	7	2.8	3	0	Trace
62	259	2	0.9	10	1	0
108	448	8	3	5	4	0.5
99	414	7	1.8	5	5	0.5
103	429	7	1.9	5	5	0.5
123	512	10	3.4	6	4	0.3
118	488	9	3.2	6	4	0.3
126	525	10	3.5	6	4	0.3
116	482	8	3	6	4	0.3
84	352	5	1.7	6	4	0.6
92	384	6	2	6	4	0.6
110	457	8	3.1	6	3	0.3
117	486	9	3.3	7	3	0.3
53	218	5	1.8	3	0	0
192	801	18	3.6	9	7	0.5

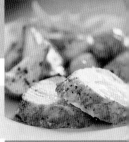

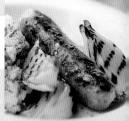

MEAT &
MEAT DISHES 43

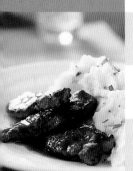

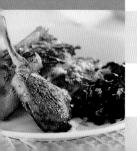

BEEFBURGERS	AVERAGE PORTION g
Beefburgers, fried	36
Beefburgers, grilled	100
Beefburgers, fried	100
Beefburgers, grilled	100
Beefburgers, low-fat, fried	100
Beefburgers, low-fat, grilled	100
Beefburgers in gravy, canned	100

PIES AND PASTIES	
Beef pie, shop bought	141
Cornish pasty	155
Cornish pasty, shop bought	155
Lamb samosa, baked	70
Lamb samosa, deep-fried	70
Pork and egg pie	60
Pork pie	60
Pork pie, mini	50
Sausage rolls, flaky pastry	60
Sausage rolls, shortcrust pastry	60
Steak and kidney pie, double crust	120
Steak and kidney pie, shop bought	141

OFFAL	
Heart, lamb, roasted	200
Heart, lamb, stewed	200
Heart, ox, stewed	200
Heart, pig, stewed	100
Kidney, lamb, fried	35
Kidney, ox, stewed	112
Kidney, pig, fried	140
Kidney, pig, stewed	140
Liver, calf, fried	100

Unless otherwise stated, all meat is lean and trimmed, and all chops and
cutlets are boned. Steaks are medium-sized. Unless stated otherwise, all
dishes are homemade.

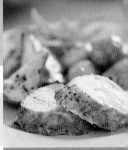

ENERGY kcal	ENERGY kJ	FAT g	SATURATED FAT g	PROTEIN g	CARBOHYDRATE g	FIBRE g
118	493	9	3.9	10	0	0
326	1355	24	10.9	27	0	0
303	1261	23	8.7	24	1	0.2
287	1194	20	8.8	25	1	0.2
193	807	11	5	24	0	0
178	745	10	4.4	23	1	0
171	713	12	4.8	12	5	Trace
437	1826	24	11.8	12	38	0.7
456	1905	28	9.8	10	43	2.6
414	1731	25	9.1	10	39	1.4
187	781	10	2.5	8	16	1.2
265	1097	22	3.3	6	12	0.8
178	740	13	4.4	6	10	0.5
228	947	18	6.8	6	11	0.5
196	815	14	5.7	5	13	0.5
238	991	17	6.5	6	15	0.8
229	953	16	5.8	6	17	0.9
406	1694	26	9.7	16	27	1.1
437	1826	24	11.8	12	38	0.7
452	1888	28	6.2	51	0	0
312	1308	15	6	24	20	0
314	1322	10	5	56	0	0
162	678	7	1.3	25	0	0
66	274	4	0.4	8	0	0
155	648	5	1.6	27	0	0
283	1187	13	2.1	41	0	0
214	897	9	2.8	34	0	0
176	734	10	2.7	22	Trace	0

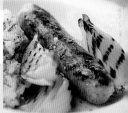

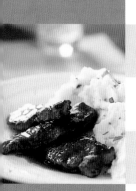

OFFAL	AVERAGE PORTION g
Liver, chicken, fried	70
Liver, lamb, fried	100
Liver, ox, stewed	70
Liver, pig, stewed	70
Liver and bacon, fried	100
Liver and onions, stewed	142
Liver sausage	40
Oxtail, stewed	260
Sweetbread, lamb, fried	100
Tongue	50
Tongue, canned	50
Tongue, ox, stewed	50
Tongue, sheep, stewed	50
Tripe and onions, stewed	100

PORK, BACON AND HAM

Bacon

Collar joint, boiled	46
Collar joint, untrimmed, boiled	46
Loin steaks, grilled	100
Rashers, back, dry-cured, grilled	100
Rashers, back, dry-fried	100
Rashers, back, grilled	100
Rashers, back, untrimmed, grilled	100
Rashers, back, grilled crispy	100
Rashers, back, reduced salt, grilled	100
Rashers, back, smoked, grilled	100
Rashers, back, sweetcure, grilled	100
Rashers, back, 'tendersweet', grilled	100
Rashers, middle, fried	100
Rashers, middle, grilled	100
Rashers, streaky, fried	100
Rashers, streaky, grilled	100

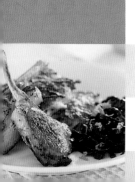

Unless otherwise stated, all meat is lean and trimmed, and all chops and
cutlets are boned. Steaks are medium-sized. Unless stated otherwise, all
dishes are homemade.

ENERGY kcal	ENERGY kJ	FAT g	SATURATED FAT g	PROTEIN g	CARBOHYDRATE g	FIBRE g
118	494	6	3.5	15	Trace	0
237	989	13	4.9	30	Trace	0
139	582	7	2.5	17	2	0
132	555	6	1.8	18	2	0
247	1030	15	2.1	29	Trace	0
210	879	11	2.1	21	8	1.4
90	377	7	2.1	5	2	0.3
632	2636	35	12	79	0	0
217	910	11	5	29	0	0
101	418	7	3	9	Trace	Trace
107	442	8	3.2	8	Trace	0
121	504	9	3	10	0	0
145	599	12	5	9	0	0
93	393	3	1.5	8	10	0.7
88	368	4	1.7	12	0	0
150	619	12	4.9	9	0	0
191	799	10	3.5	26	0	0
257	1071	16	6	28	0	0
295	1225	22	8.3	24	0	0
214	892	12	4.6	26	0	0
287	1194	22	8.1	23	0	0
313	1308	19	7.1	36	0	0
282	1172	21	7.8	24	0	0
293	1216	22	8.3	23	0	0
258	1074	17	6.6	24	2	0
213	889	12	4.5	26	Trace	0
350	1452	29	9.8	23	0	0
307	1276	23	8.4	25	0	0
335	1389	27	9.1	24	0	0
337	1400	27	9.8	24	0	0

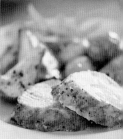

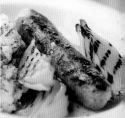

PORK, BACON AND HAM	AVERAGE PORTION g
Belly joint, untrimmed, roasted	110
Belly, untrimmed, grilled	110
Chump chops, untrimmed, fried	170
Chump steaks, untrimmed, fried	170
Crackling, cooked	50
Fillet, grilled, lean	120
Fillet, untrimmed, grilled	120
Fillet strips, stir-fried, lean	90
Gammon	
Joint, boiled	170
Rashers, grilled	100
Ham	
Ham, canned	90
Ham, Parma	47
Ham, premium	56
Pork shoulder, cured	100
Kebabs, grilled	90
Kebabs, untrimmed, grilled	90
Leg joint, untrimmed, frozen, roasted	90
Leg joint, roasted medium	90
Leg joint, untrimmed, roasted medium	90
Leg joint, roasted well done	90
Leg joint, untrimmed, roasted well done	90
Loin chops, grilled	75
Loin chops, untrimmed, grilled	75
Loin chops, grilled	120
Loin chops, untrimmed, grilled	120
Loin chops, roasted	75
Loin chops, untrimmed, roasted	75
Loin joint, pot roasted	90
Loin joint, untrimmed, pot roasted	90
Loin joint, roasted	90
Loin joint, untrimmed, roasted	90
Loin steaks, fried	120

Unless otherwise stated, all meat is lean and trimmed, and all chops and
cutlets are boned. Steaks are medium-sized. Unless stated otherwise, all
dishes are homemade.

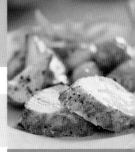

ENERGY kcal	ENERGY kJ	FAT g	SATURATED FAT g	PROTEIN g	CARBOHYDRATE g	FIBRE g
322	1341	24	8.1	28	0	0
352	1465	26	9	30	0	0
498	2069	37	11.9	42	0	0
369	1542	20	6.3	47	0	0
275	1140	23	7.7	18	0	0
204	863	5	1.8	40	0	0
214	899	6	2.3	40	0	0
164	688	5	1.2	29	0	0
347	1447	21	7	40	0	0
199	834	10	3.4	28	0	0
96	404	4	1.4	15	0	0
105	438	6	2	13	Trace	Trace
74	310	3	1	12	0	0
103	435	4	1.2	17	1	0
161	679	4	1.4	31	0	0
170	717	5	2	30	0	0
202	842	10	3.6	28	0	0
164	689	5	1.7	30	0	0
194	813	9	3.2	28	0	0
167	701	5	1.6	31	0	0
233	974	14	4.9	27	0	0
140	585	5	1.8	23	0	0
191	800	12	4.3	21	0	0
221	929	8	2.6	38	0	0
308	1289	19	6.7	35	0	0
181	758	8	2.8	28	0	0
226	942	14	5.3	24	0	0
177	744	7	2.6	28	0	0
275	1142	21	7.4	22	0	0
164	687	6	2.2	27	0	0
228	949	15	5.3	24	0	0
229	962	9	2.8	38	0	0

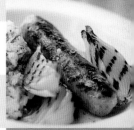

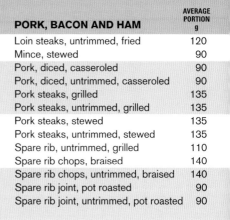

PORK, BACON AND HAM	AVERAGE PORTION g
Loin steaks, untrimmed, fried	120
Mince, stewed	90
Pork, diced, casseroled	90
Pork, diced, untrimmed, casseroled	90
Pork steaks, grilled	135
Pork steaks, untrimmed, grilled	135
Pork steaks, stewed	135
Pork steaks, untrimmed, stewed	135
Spare rib, untrimmed, grilled	110
Spare rib chops, braised	140
Spare rib chops, untrimmed, braised	140
Spare rib joint, pot roasted	90
Spare rib joint, untrimmed, pot roasted	90

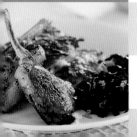

Unless otherwise stated, all meat is lean and trimmed, and all chops and
cutlets are boned. Steaks are medium-sized. Unless stated otherwise, all
dishes are homemade.

ENERGY kcal	ENERGY kJ	FAT g	SATURATED FAT g	PROTEIN g	CARBOHYDRATE g	FIBRE g
331	1378	22	7.2	33	0	0
172	720	9	3.5	22	0	0
166	698	6	1.7	29	0	0
166	698	6	1.8	28	0	0
228	963	5	1.8	46	0	0
267	1123	10	3.6	44	0	0
238	1000	6	1.8	45	0	0
269	1126	11	3.2	42	0	0
321	1340	21	8.3	32	0	0
298	1249	14	5	43	0	0
346	1446	21	7.7	39	0	0
181	759	8	2.9	27	0	0
234	973	16	6	22	0	0

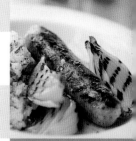

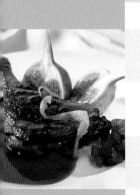

CHICKEN

	AVERAGE PORTION g
Breast, casseroled	130
Breast, skinned, casseroled	130
Breast, grilled	130
Breast, grilled and skinned	130
Breast, skinned, grilled	130
Breast strips, stir-fried	90
Corn-fed chicken, roasted, dark meat	90
Corn-fed chicken, roasted, light meat	90
Dark meat, roasted	100
Drumsticks, casseroled	47
Drumsticks, skinned, casseroled	47
Drumsticks, roasted	47
Drumsticks, skinned, roasted	47
Leg quarter, casseroled	146
Leg quarter, skinned, casseroled	146
Leg quarter, roasted	146
Light meat, roasted	100
Thighs, casseroled	45
Thighs, skinned, boned and diced, casseroled	45
Wing quarter, casseroled	150
Wing quarter, skinned, casseroled	150
Wing quarter, roasted	150
Wings, grilled	100

CHICKEN PRODUCTS

Chicken fingers, baked	90
Chicken goujons, baked	90
Chicken in crumbs, stuffed with cheese and vegetables, baked	100
Chicken in white sauce, canned	100
Chicken Kiev, frozen, baked	170

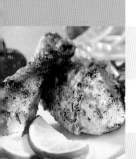

Unless otherwise stated, chicken and turkey are neither skinned nor boned, game is skinned and trimmed and dishes are homemade.

ENERGY kcal	ENERGY kJ	FAT g	SATURATED FAT g	PROTEIN g	CARBOHYDRATE g	FIBRE g
239	1004	11	3.1	35	0	0
148	628	7	2	37	0	0
225	946	8	1.2	38	0	0
191	807	4	1.2	39	0	0
192	814	4	0.8	42	0	0
145	609	4	0.8	27	0	0
167	695	9	2.5	22	0	0
127	536	4	1.1	23	0	0
196	819	11	2.9	24	0	0
102	425	7	1.8	10	0	0
87	363	5	1.2	11	0	0
87	364	4	1.2	12	0	0
71	301	2	0.7	13	0	0
317	1320	20	5.5	33	0	0
257	1075	12	3.4	37	0	0
345	1432	25	6.7	31	0	0
153	645	4	1	30	0	0
105	436	7	2	10	0	0
81	340	4	1.1	12	0	0
315	1316	19	5.3	37	0	0
246	1035	9	2.6	40	0	0
339	1415	21	5.9	37	0	0
274	1146	17	4.6	27	Trace	0
185	774	9	2.7	11	17	Trace
249	1045	13	3.6	17	18	0.6
230	963	14	4.1	16	11	0.9
141	590	8	2.3	14	3	Trace
456	1902	29	12.1	32	19	1

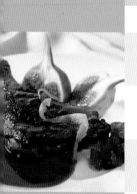

CHICKEN PRODUCTS	AVERAGE PORTION g
Chicken pancakes, frozen, shallow-fried	100
Chicken roll	24
Chicken slices	80

CHICKEN PIES

Chicken and mushroom pie, single crust	100
Chicken pie, individual, baked	130

CHICKEN DISHES

Chicken chasseur	260
Chicken in sauce with vegetables	290
Chicken curry	350
Chicken curry, with bone	350
Chicken curry, without bone	300
Chicken fricassée	200
Chicken in white sauce, made with semi-skimmed milk	200
Chicken in white sauce, made with whole milk	200
Chicken risotto	350
Coronation chicken	200
Lemon chicken	100
Tandoori chicken	100

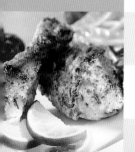

Unless otherwise stated, chicken and turkey are neither skinned nor boned, game is skinned and trimmed and dishes are homemade.

ENERGY kcal	ENERGY kJ	FAT g	SATURATED FAT g	PROTEIN g	CARBOHYDRATE g	FIBRE g
260	1090	14	1.4	6	29	0.1
31	132	1	0.4	4	1	Trace
91	386	1	0.3	19	2	0
200	836	10	4.5	13	14	0.6
374	1563	21	9.1	12	32	1
203	861	5	0.8	33	7	0.8
336	1412	15	7	39	13	0.9
522	2174	31	14	42	19	4.5
539	2237	44	6	27	8	2.4
615	2550	51	6.6	31	9	2.7
214	896	12	4.8	22	6	1
310	1298	16	5	34	10	0.2
328	1376	18	6.2	34	10	0.2
546	2310	10	4.5	31	84	Trace
728	3012	63	10.4	33	6	Trace
155	652	6	0.8	16	9	Trace
214	897	11	3.3	27	2	Trace

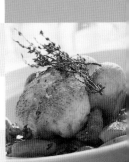

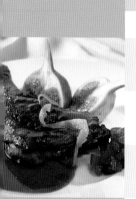

	AVERAGE PORTION g
GAME	
Duck, roasted	185
Duck, untrimmed, roasted	185
Goose, roasted	185
Goose, untrimmed, roasted	185
Grouse, roasted	160
Pheasant, roasted	160
Pigeon, roasted	115
Rabbit, stewed	160
Venison, roasted	120
TURKEY	
Breast, grilled and skinned	90
Dark meat, roasted	90
Drumsticks, roasted	90
Drumsticks, roasted and skinned	90
Light meat, from self-basting bird, roasted	90
Light meat, roasted	90
Mince, stewed	90
Strips, stir-fried	90
Thighs, diced, skinned, boned, casseroled	90

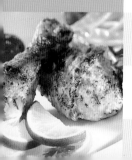

Unless otherwise stated, chicken and turkey are neither skinned nor boned, game is skinned and trimmed and dishes are homemade.

ENERGY kcal	ENERGY kJ	FAT g	SATURATED FAT g	PROTEIN g	CARBOHYDRATE g	FIBRE g
361	1508	19	6.1	47	0	0
783	3238	92	21.1	37	0	0
590	2455	41	13.7	54	0	0
557	2316	39	12.2	51	0	0
205	869	3	0.8	44	0	0
352	1469	5	0.6	45	0	0
215	903	9	3	33	0	0
182	766	5	2.7	34	0	0
198	838	3	1	43	0	0
140	592	2	0.5	32	0	0
159	671	6	1.8	26	0	0
167	702	8	2.3	25	0	0
146	615	5	1.5	25	0	0
147	619	4	1.1	29	0	0
138	583	2	0.6	30	0	0
158	665	6	1.8	26	0	0
148	623	4	1.1	28	0	0
163	684	7	2.3	25	0	0

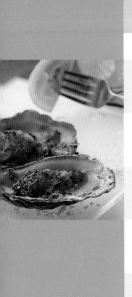

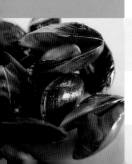

FISH	AVERAGE PORTION g
Anchovies, canned in oil	10
Cod, baked	120
Cod, coated in batter, frozen, baked	180
Cod, coated in crumbs, frozen, fried	100
Cod, dried, salted, boiled	90
Cod, frozen, grilled	120
Cod, in batter, fried	180
Cod, in parsley sauce, frozen, boiled	170
Cod, poached	120
Cod, smoked, poached	120
Cod, steamed	120
Conger eel, grilled	115
Dogfish, in batter, fried	125
Eels, jellied	70
Eels, stewed	70
Haddock, grilled	120
Haddock, in batter, fried	120
Haddock, in crumbs, fried	120
Haddock, in crumbs, frozen, fried	120
Haddock, in flour, fried	120
Haddock, poached	120
Haddock, smoked, poached	150
Haddock, smoked, steamed	150
Haddock, steamed	120
Hake, grilled	100
Halibut, grilled	145
Halibut, poached	110
Halibut, steamed	110
Herring, grilled	119
Herring, in oatmeal, fried	119
Herring, pickled	90
Hoki, grilled	190
Kipper, baked	130

Unless otherwise stated, values for bottled and canned seafood are for drained weights.

ENERGY kcal	ENERGY kJ	FAT g	SATURATED FAT g	PROTEIN g	CARBOHYDRATE g	FIBRE g
28	117	2	0.4	3	0	0
115	490	1	0.4	26	Trace	0
380	1589	21	6.5	23	26	1.1
235	983	14	1.5	12	15	0.4
124	527	1	0.2	29	0	0
114	482	2	0.5	25	Trace	0
445	1856	28	7.4	29	21	0.9
143	598	5	3	20	5	0.2
113	475	1	0.4	25	Trace	0
121	511	2	0.7	26	Trace	0
100	420	1	0.2	22	0	0
158	660	6	Trace	25	0	0
369	1531	27	6.6	18	13	0.5
69	284	5	1.3	6	Trace	0
141	589	9	1.3	14	0	0
125	530	1	0.2	29	0	0
278	1163	17	4.4	21	12	0.5
209	875	10	0.8	26	4	0.2
235	986	12	1	18	15	0.7
166	698	5	0.5	25	5	0.2
136	572	5	3.1	21	1	0
201	843	9	5.6	28	2	0
152	644	1	0.3	35	0	0
107	454	1	0.1	25	0	0
113	478	3	0.4	22	0	0
175	744	3	0.6	37	0	0
169	713	6	3	27	1	0
144	608	4	0.6	26	0	0
215	900	13	3.3	24	0	0
278	1160	18	3.3	27	2	0.1
188	789	10	3.3	15	9	0
230	969	5	1	46	0	0
267	1112	15	2.3	33	0	0

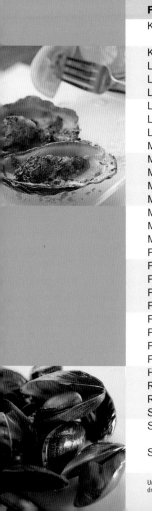

FISH	AVERAGE PORTION g
Kipper, boil-in-the-bag, boiled, with butter added	170
Kipper, grilled	130
Lemon sole, goujons, baked	170
Lemon sole, goujons, fried	170
Lemon sole, grilled	109
Lemon sole, in crumbs, fried	109
Lemon sole, steamed	109
Lobster, boiled, dressed with shell	250
Mackerel, canned in brine	200
Mackerel, canned in tomato sauce	125
Mackerel, fried	161
Mackerel, grilled	147
Mackerel, smoked	150
Monkfish, grilled	70
Mullet, Grey, grilled	100
Mullet, Red, grilled	110
Pilchards, canned in tomato sauce	215
Plaice, frozen, grilled	165
Plaice, frozen, steamed	130
Plaice, goujons, baked	130
Plaice, goujons, fried	150
Plaice, grilled	130
Plaice, in batter, fried	200
Plaice, in crumbs, fried	150
Plaice, in crumbs, frozen, fried	150
Plaice, steamed	130
Red snapper, fried	102
Rock salmon, in batter, fried	125
Salmon, grilled	82
Salmon, pink, canned in brine, skinned and boned	100
Salmon, raw	100

Unless otherwise stated, values for bottled and canned seafood are for drained weights.

ENERGY kcal	ENERGY kJ	FAT g	SATURATED FAT g	PROTEIN g	CARBOHYDRATE g	FIBRE g
403	1673	30	2.7	34	Trace	0
332	1378	25	4	26	0	0
318	1318	25	Trace	27	25	Trace
636	2640	49	5.4	26	24	Trace
106	445	2	0.2	22	0	0
235	985	14	1.4	18	10	0.4
99	419	1	0.1	22	0	0
258	1088	4	0.5	55	Trace	0
474	1970	36	8	38	0	0
258	1070	19	4.1	20	2	Trace
438	1819	31	6.4	39	0	0
351	1461	25	5.1	31	0	0
531	2198	46	9.5	28	0	0
67	285	0	0.1	16	0	0
150	629	5	1.4	26	0	0
133	561	5	1.4	22	0	0
310	1292	17	3.7	36	2	Trace
200	843	3	0.5	42	0	0
120	506	2	0.3	25	0	0
395	1651	24	0	11	36	Trace
639	2657	48	5.4	13	41	Trace
125	525	2	0.4	26	0	0
514	2144	34	9	30	24	1
342	1427	21	2.3	27	13	0.3
261	1094	14	1.5	21	14	0.5
121	510	2	0.4	25	0	0
129	542	3	0.7	25	0	0
369	1531	27	6.6	18	13	0.5
176	735	11	2.1	20	0	0
153	644	7	1.3	24	0	0
180	750	11	1.9	20	0	0

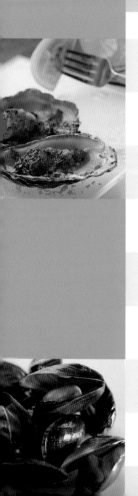

FISH	AVERAGE PORTION g
Salmon, red, canned in brine, skinned and boned	100
Salmon, smoked	56
Salmon, steamed	77
Sardines, canned in brine	100
Sardines, canned in oil	100
Sardines, canned in tomato sauce	100
Sardines, grilled	40
Skate, grilled	215
Skate, in batter, fried	170
Sprats, fried	132
Swordfish, grilled	125
Trout, brown, steamed	155
Trout, rainbow, grilled	155
Tuna, canned in brine	45
Tuna, canned in oil	45
Tuna, raw	45
Whitebait, in flour, fried	80
Whiting, in crumbs, fried	162
Whiting, steamed	85

FISH PRODUCTS AND DISHES

Caviare, bottled in brine	19
Fish balls, steamed	50
Fish cakes, fried	100
Fish cakes, grilled	100
Fish cakes, salmon, grilled	100
Fish fingers, cod, fried	56
Fish fingers, cod, grilled	56
Fish paste	10
Fisherman's pie, shop bought	170
Kedgeree	300
Mackerel pâté, smoked	40

Unless otherwise stated, values for bottled and canned seafood are for drained weights. Dishes are homemade unless otherwise stated.

ENERGY kcal	ENERGY kJ	FAT g	SATURATED FAT g	PROTEIN g	CARBOHYDRATE g	FIBRE g
167	700	8	1.7	22	0	0
80	335	3	0.4	14	0	0
152	634	10	1.8	15	0	0
172	721	10	2.8	22	0	0
220	918	14	2.9	23	0	0
162	678	10	2.8	17	1	Trace
78	326	4	1.2	10	0	0
170	725	1	0.2	41	0	0
286	1193	17	4.3	25	8	0.3
548	2268	46	7	33	0	0
174	729	6	1.5	29	0	0
209	877	7	1.6	36	0	0
209	876	8	1.7	33	0	0
45	190	1	0.1	11	0	0
85	357	4	0.7	12	0	0
61	258	2	0.5	11	0	0
420	1739	38	2.1	16	4	0.2
309	1298	17	1.8	29	11	0.3
78	331	1	0.1	18	0	0
17	73	1	0.2	2	0	0
37	157	0	0.9	6	3	0
218	912	14	1.4	8	16	0.6
154	650	5	0.6	10	20	0.6
273	1137	20	2.9	10	14	0.7
133	557	8	2	7	9	0.3
112	469	5	1.6	8	9	0.4
17	71	1	0.5	2	0	0
201	838	9	3.1	15	15	0.9
498	2103	24	6.9	43	32	Trace
147	608	14	2.5	5	1	Trace

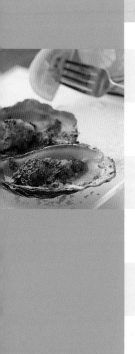

FISH PRODUCTS AND DISHES	AVERAGE PORTION g
Roe, cod, hard, coated in batter, fried	160
Roe, cod, hard, fried	116
Roe, herring, soft, fried	85
Salmon en croûte, shop bought	100
Taramasalata	45
Tuna pâté	40

SEAFOOD AND SHELLFISH

Cockles, boiled	25
Cockles, bottled in vinegar	25
Crab, boiled, dressed with shell	130
Crab, canned in brine	40
Lobster, boiled, dressed with shell	250
Mussels, boiled and shelled	40
Mussels, canned or bottled without shells	40
Oysters, uncooked and shelled	120
Prawns, boiled and shelled	60
Scallops, steamed and shelled	70
Squid, in batter, fried	120
Whelks, boiled and shelled	30
Winkles, boiled and shelled	30

SEAFOOD PRODUCTS AND DISHES

Crabsticks	100
Scampi, in breadcrumbs, frozen, fried	170
Seafood cocktail	88
Seafood pasta, shop bought	290

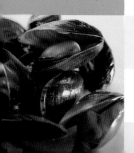

Unless otherwise stated, values for bottled and canned seafood are for drained weights. Dishes are homemade unless otherwise stated.

ENERGY kcal	ENERGY kJ	FAT g	SATURATED FAT g	PROTEIN g	CARBOHYDRATE g	FIBRE g
302	1264	19	2.6	20	14	0.3
234	979	14	1.9	24	3	0.1
225	941	13	2.2	22	4	0.2
288	1202	19	3.1	12	18	0.3
227	935	24	1.8	1	2	Trace
94	393	7	3.1	7	0	Trace
13	57	1	0.1	3	Trace	0
15	63	1	0.1	3	Trace	0
166	696	7	0.9	25	Trace	0
31	130	0	0	7	Trace	0
258	1088	4	0.5	55	Trace	0
42	176	1	0.2	7	1	0
39	166	1	0.2	7	1	0
78	330	2	0.2	13	3	0
59	251	1	0.1	14	0	0
83	351	1	0.3	16	2	Trace
234	978	12	2.5	14	19	0.6
27	113	1	0.1	6	Trace	0
22	92	1	0.1	5	Trace	0
68	290	0	0	10	7	0
403	1685	23	2.4	16	35	0
77	325	1	0.3	14	3	0
319	1334	14	8.1	26	22	1.2

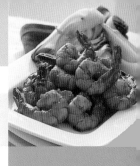

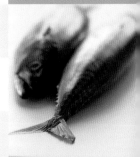

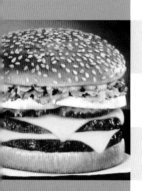

BURGER KING	AVERAGE PORTION g
Bacon and Egg Sandwich	139
Big King®	202
BK Chicken Flamer	162
BK Spicy Beanburger	239
Cajun Chicken Deli Wrap	208
Cheeseburger	129
Chicken Caesar Deli Wrap	208
Chicken Royale	210
Chicken Royale Club	241
Chicken Whopper	260
Chicken Whopper Junior	159
Chicken Whopper Lite	161
Double Cheeseburger	185
Double Cheeseburger with Bacon	195
Hamburger	117
Hash Browns, large	102
Hash Browns, medium	68
Kids Cheeseburger	120
Kids Hamburger	107
Kids Veggie Burger	165
King Fries, large	142
King Fries, regular	116
King Fries, small	74
Onion Rings, large	120
Onion Rings, regular	90
Sausage and Egg Sandwich	160
Sausage, Bacon and Egg Sandwich	182
Veggie Burger	223
Whopper®	267
Whopper Junior	151
Whopper Junior with Cheese	163
Whopper with Cheese	292
XL Double Whopper	348
XL Double Whopper with Cheese	373

Information copyright © Burger King

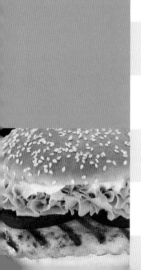

ENERGY kcal	ENERGY kJ	FAT g	SATURATED FAT g	PROTEIN g	CARBOHYDRATE g	FIBRE g
296	1153	13	3.7	15	30	2.7
540	2163	31.3	12.8	33.3	30.3	2.2
308	1295	12	2.3	20	30	3.1
505	2112	20	5.8	19	63	9.3
511	2146	27.5	3.9	18	48	3.1
331	1289	14	6.4	20	30	1.8
835	1682	25.5	3.9	18.3	45.5	3.0
638	2696	40	1.4	25	47	4.9
668	2823	42.1	2.4	26.9	47.7	5.3
548	2300	23.4	1.3	39.4	45	2.5
339	1425	13.9	0.7	24.3	29.3	1.7
289	1223	7.5	1.1	25	29.9	1.7
492	1961	26	12.4	33	30	2.1
509	2034	28.3	13.3	37.4	30.7	2.1
290	1120	11	4.2	17	30	1.8
318	1330	19.7	4.4	2.2	33.0	3.8
212	887	13	2.9	2	22	2.6
328	1276	14	6.4	19.4	29.9	1.7
287	1107	10.6	4.2	17	29.7	1.7
359	1512	11.1	1.1	11.9	52.8	7.1
490	2047	19.6	3.4	3.7	52.7	3.6
400	1672	16	2.8	3	43	2.9
259	1081	10.2	1.8	1.9	32.3	1.9
348	1458	16.7	1.9	5.8	43.7	4.6
261	1094	13	1.4	4	33	3.4
375	1481	19	5.5	20	32	3
430	1712	23.1	7.4	24.1	31.8	3.1
432	1818	17	3.5	15	55	7.6
646	2583	38	8.1	31	48	3.6
372	1475	19.6	4.4	17.4	30.6	2.1
413	1644	23	6.6	19.8	30.7	2.1
728	2921	44.7	12.5	35.4	47.9	3.6
873	3531	53.9	15.2	51.6	47.6	4.2
955	3869	60.7	19.6	56.4	47.9	4.2

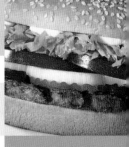

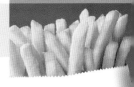

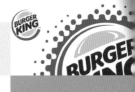

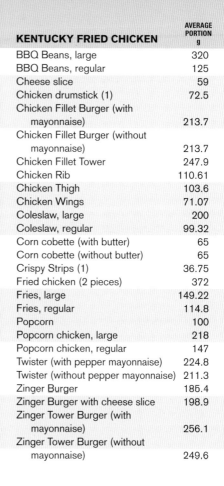

KENTUCKY FRIED CHICKEN	AVERAGE PORTION g
BBQ Beans, large	320
BBQ Beans, regular	125
Cheese slice	59
Chicken drumstick (1)	72.5
Chicken Fillet Burger (with mayonnaise)	213.7
Chicken Fillet Burger (without mayonnaise)	213.7
Chicken Fillet Tower	247.9
Chicken Rib	110.61
Chicken Thigh	103.6
Chicken Wings	71.07
Coleslaw, large	200
Coleslaw, regular	99.32
Corn cobette (with butter)	65
Corn cobette (without butter)	65
Crispy Strips (1)	36.75
Fried chicken (2 pieces)	372
Fries, large	149.22
Fries, regular	114.8
Popcorn	100
Popcorn chicken, large	218
Popcorn chicken, regular	147
Twister (with pepper mayonnaise)	224.8
Twister (without pepper mayonnaise)	211.3
Zinger Burger	185.4
Zinger Burger with cheese slice	198.9
Zinger Tower Burger (with mayonnaise)	256.1
Zinger Tower Burger (without mayonnaise)	249.6

ENERGY kcal	ENERGY kJ	FAT g	SATURATED FAT g	PROTEIN g	CARBOHYDRATE g	FIBRE g
294.4	1231.8	1.12	0.224	13.92	56.96	9.21
115	481.17	0.42	0.084	5.22	21.36	4.14
194.1	807	15.39	10.66	11.21	1.062	0
185	775	11.25	1.91	13.96	7.17	0.8
470.85	1976.02	19.6	3.06	31.99	41.52	3.38
408.94	1716	17.06	2.64	27.78	36.07	2.94
574.3	2406	27.82	5.6	27.78	49.02	3.6
292	1222	17.21	2.38	24.13	10.02	1.16
288	1199	20.35	4.27	19.92	5.8	0.87
574.3	2406	27.82	5.6	27.78	49.02	3.6
294	1212	26.9	1.6	1.86	10.92	2.66
146	606	13.45	0.8	0.93	5.46	1.33
68.68	290	1.69	0.76	2.13	11.27	1.40
79.7	336.96	1.5	0	2.66	14.77	3.05
113.23	472.92	6.37	0.98	7.63	6.11	0.61
1551	2305.43	23	3.8	28	14	0.8
382	1600	19.22	4.46	4.95	47.38	3.97
294	1232	14.78	3.43	3.81	36.44	3.06
264.5	1104.75	16.075	2.35	17.25	12.75	1.025
573.97	2397.31	35	4.95	37.5	27.62	1.06
388.82	1623.98	24	3.35	25.4	18.71	0.72
541.37	2262	30.02	6.26	23.5	43.88	4.14
499.51	2090	29.07	6.07	22.77	42.49	4.00
440	1847	19.33	2.89	25.49	41.05	2.56
490.60	2055.92	19.6	5.37	26.11	41.82	2.59
607.29	2546	31.24	6.65	30.99	50.62	3.17
555.51	2324.31	25.5	6.81	31.68	51.73	3.25

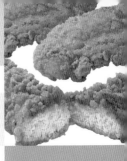

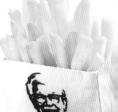

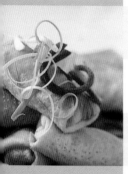

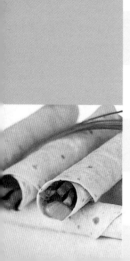

INDIAN DISHES

	AVERAGE PORTION g
Chicken biryani	400
Chicken dhansak	350
Chicken dupiaza	350
Chicken jalfrezi	350
Chicken korma	350
Chicken tikka	350
Chicken tikka masala	350
Lamb balti	350
Lamb rogan josh	350
Meat samosas	70
Poppadoms	70
Prawn bhuna	400
Prawn madras	350
Vegetable balti	350
Vegetable biryani	350

ORIENTAL DISHES

Aromatic crispy duck	125
Chicken chop suey	450
Chicken chow mein	350
Chicken fried rice	350
Chicken satay	170
Chicken with cashew nuts	360
Egg fried rice	270
Green chicken curry	350
Meat spring roll	55
Pancakes	70
Prawn crackers	70
Sesame prawn toasts	70
Spare ribs	340
Stir-fried beef with green peppers in black bean sauce	360
Stir-fried Thai vegetable curry	350

ENERGY kcals	ENERGY kJ	FAT g	SATURATED FAT g	PROTEIN g	CARBOHYDRATE g	FIBRE g
651	2144	30	8.0	34	66	4.4
503	1509	30	6.0	40	21	6.7
397	1168	25	4.9	40	4	6.3
416	1203	27	5.3	34	11	7.0
668	1753	51	20.0	44	8	7.0
421	1470	15	5.6	71	Trace	1.0
551	1488	40	13.7	47	Trace	7.7
534	1518	35	8.8	43	11	6.7
510	1422	35	9.8	43	6	3.1
191	553	12	3.2	8	13	1.5
351	916	27	5.6	8	20	4.1
363	802	35	4.0	6	7	7.6
390	1042	29	3.5	27	6	7.0
373	983	28	5.3	8	23	7.7
467	1468	25	4.9	10	55	6.0
412	1107	30	9.1	35	15	1.1
363	1095	21	3.6	37	7	5.4
516	1662	25	4.2	30	46	3.9
562	1948	21	3.5	23	75	0.0
324	1006	18	4.9	37	5	3.7
470	1331	31	5.4	38	10	0.0
491	1809	13	1.6	12	87	2.2
417	1125	30	18.2	31	5	8.4
133	374	9	2.1	4	10	1.0
213	790	6	Trace	6	37	0.0
386	1061	27	2.6	0	37	0.8
268	699	21	2.7	9	12	1.3
873	2358	64	10.2	75	7	1.0
373	1158	20	5.0	38	11	6.5
351	882	29	13.7	13	11	9.1

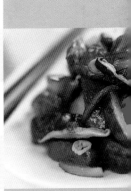

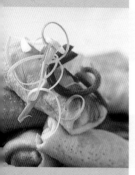

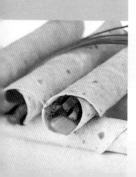

ORIENTAL DISHES	AVERAGE PORTION g
Stir-fried vegetables	340
Sweet and sour chicken	300
Sweet and sour pork, battered	300
Szechuan prawns with vegetables	350

BURGERS AND HOTDOGS

Cheeseburger, large, double	258
Cheeseburger, large, single	219
Cheeseburger, regular, double	228
Cheeseburger, triple, plain	304
Hamburger, large, double	226
Hamburger, large, single, with seasoning and sauce	172
Hamburger, large, triple patty, seasoning and sauce	259
Hamburger, regular, double, plain	176
Hamburger, regular, double, with seasoning and sauce	215
Hamburger, regular, single, plain	90
Hamburger, regular, single, with seasoning and sauce	106

MEXICAN DISHES

Burrito, beans	217
Burrito, beans and cheese	186
Burrito, beans and chilli peppers	204
Burrito, beans and meat	231
Burrito, beans, cheese and beef	203
Burrito, beef	220
Burrito, beef and chilli peppers	201
Burrito, beef, cheese and chilli peppers	304
Chimichanga, beef	174

Unless otherwise specified, burgers include garnish, seasonings and sauce.

ENERGY kcals	ENERGY kJ	FAT g	SATURATED FAT g	PROTEIN g	CARBOHYDRATE g	FIBRE g
177	455	14	2.4	6	7	6.1
575	1810	30	3.9	23	57	1.8
705	2115	42	6.9	23	63	3.0
297	912	16	1.8	27	11	4.9
704	2946	44	17.7	38	40	2.1
563	2354	33	15	28	38	2.1
650	2718	35	12.8	30	53	2.1
796	3332	51	21.7	56	27	2.1
540	2260	27	10.5	34	40	2.1
427	1785	21	7.9	23	37	2.1
692	2893	41	15.9	50	29	2.1
544	2276	28	10.4	30	43	2
576	2410	32	12	32	39	2.1
274	1148	12	4.1	12	31	2
272	1140	10	3.6	12	34	2.3
447	1871	13	6.9	14	71	1.5
378	1579	12	6.8	15	55	1.5
412	1724	15	7.6	16	58	1.5
508	2125	18	8.3	22	66	1.5
331	1384	13	7.1	15	40	1.5
524	2191	21	10.5	27	59	1.5
426	1783	17	8	22	49	1.5
632	2645	25	10.4	41	64	1.5
425	1777	20	8.5	20	43	1.5

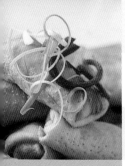

MEXICAN DISHES

	AVERAGE PORTION g
Chimichanga, beef and cheese	183
Chimichanga, beef and chilli peppers	190
Chimichanga, beef, cheese and chilli peppers	180
Enchilada, cheese	163
Enchilada, cheese and beef	192
Enchilada, vegetable	360
Fajita, chicken, meat only	170
Nachos, cheese	113
Nachos, cheese and jalapeno peppers	204
Nachos, cheese, beans, ground beef and peppers	255

PIZZA

Pizza, cheese and tomato, deep pan, shop bought	220
Pizza, cheese and tomato, deep pan	220
Pizza, cheese and tomato, French bread, frozen, shop bought	200
Pizza, cheese and tomato, frozen, shop bought	200
Pizza, cheese and tomato, thin base	116
Pizza, chicken, deep pan, shop bought	230
Pizza, fish topped, deep pan	230
Pizza, fish topped, thin base	150
Pizza, ham and pineapple, shop bought	200
Pizza, meat topped, deep pan	230
Pizza, meat topped, frozen, shop bought	200
Pizza, meat topped, thin base	150
Pizza, meat, deep pan, shop bought	230
Pizza, vegetable topped, deep pan	290
Pizza, vegetable topped, thin base	150

Unless otherwise specified, pizzas are takeaway.

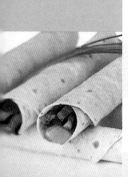

ENERGY kcals	ENERGY kJ	FAT g	SATURATED FAT g	PROTEIN g	CARBOHYDRATE g	FIBRE g
443	1854	23	11.2	20	39	1.5
424	1773	19	8.3	18	46	1.5
364	1521	18	8.4	15	38	1.5
319	1337	19	10.6	10	29	1
323	1350	18	9	12	30	1
525	1690	26	7.6	23	54	7.6
213	676	11	3.6	29	1	1.7
438	1208	31	11.6	18	24	3.4
608	2544	34	14	17	60	2
569	2379	31	12.5	20	56	2
471	1987	15	7.7	24	64	4.8
547	2310	16	11.4	27	77	4.8
461	1942	16	6.6	21	63	3.8
475	2002	18	9	23	60	3.8
322	1355	12	9.3	17	39	2.2
565	2382	19	7.8	31	72	4.6
507	2138	16	6.2	30	64	4.6
343	1446	12	9.2	20	41	2.8
521	2196	17	6.8	27	69	4.8
557	2345	21	14	30	67	4.6
496	2087	19	7.6	23	61	3.8
391	1642	18	7.5	21	39	2.8
624	2624	25	9.7	32	73	4.8
621	2624	18	7.8	32	88	4.9
332	1398	11	4.1	16	44	2.8

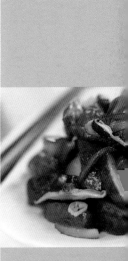

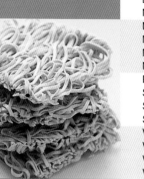

RICE, PASTA AND NOODLES	AVERAGE PORTION g
Brown rice, boiled	180
Macaroni, boiled	230
Macaroni, wholemeal, boiled	230
Noodles, egg, boiled	230
Noodles, boiled	230
Noodles, fried	230
Red rice, boiled	230
Savoury rice, cooked	180
Spaghetti, boiled	220
Spaghetti, wholemeal, boiled	230
White rice, easy cook, boiled	180
White rice, fried in lard/dripping	300
White rice, glutinous, boiled	230
White rice, polished, boiled	230

RICE AND PASTA DISHES

Cannelloni, meat, shop bought	260
Cannelloni, spinach	340
Cannelloni, vegetable	340
Chicken risotto	340
Lasagne, meat, shop bought	420
Lasagne, spinach	420
Lasagne, spinach, wholemeal	420
Lasagne, vegetable	420
Lasagne, vegetable, wholemeal	420
Pasta with ham and mushroom sauce	235
Pasta with meat and tomato sauce	235
Peppers, stuffed with rice	175
Pilau, mushroom	180
Pilau, vegetable	180
Ravioli, stuffed with cheese, tomato and herbs, shop bought	250

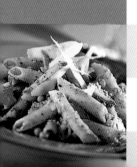

Unless otherwise stated, all dishes are homemade.

ENERGY kcal	ENERGY kJ	FAT g	SATURATED FAT g	PROTEIN g	CARBOHYDRATE g	FIBRE g
254	1075	2	0.5	5	58	1.4
198	840	1	0.2	7	43	2.1
198	840	1	0.2	7	43	6.4
143	607	1	0.2	5	30	1.4
143	607	1	0.2	6	30	1.6
352	1467	26	1	4	26	1.2
184	784	1	0.2	4	43	1.4
256	1078	6	2	5	47	2.5
229	972	2	0.2	8	49	2.6
260	1116	2	0.2	11	53	8.1
248	1057	2	0.5	5	56	0.2
393	1662	10	4.2	7	75	1.8
150	633	1	0.2	4	34	0.5
283	1201	1	0.2	5	68	0.5
315	1326	13	5.2	17	35	3.1
449	1880	26	7.8	15	43	2.7
493	2067	31	11.6	15	43	2.4
546	2310	10	4.5	31	84	Trace
601	2533	26	11.8	31	66	2.9
365	1541	13	5.5	15	53	4.6
391	1659	13	5.5	18	55	9.7
428	1810	18	9.2	17	52	4.2
445	1877	19	9.2	20	52	8.8
284	1194	14	8.2	13	27	2.1
263	1102	10	4	16	30	2
149	630	4	0.7	3	27	2.3
248	1048	8	4.5	4	43	0.7
248	1053	8	4.3	5	43	1
304	1267	13	7.9	17	30	0.6

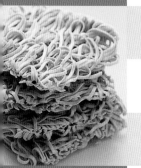

RICE AND PASTA DISHES	AVERAGE PORTION g
Ravioli, stuffed with meat and vegetables, shop bought	250
Rice and blackeye beans	200
Rice and blackeye beans, brown rice	200
Risotto, chicken	340
Risotto, vegetable, brown rice	290
Risotto, vegetable	290
Spaghetti bolognese, shop bought	400
Tortellini, stuffed with cheese and ham, shop bought	250
Vine leaves, stuffed with rice	80

Unless otherwise stated, all dishes are homemade.

ENERGY kcal	ENERGY kJ	FAT g	SATURATED FAT g	PROTEIN g	CARBOHYDRATE g	FIBRE g
324	1350	15	8.9	16	34	3.4
366	1556	7	3	12	68	2.8
350	1488	7	3	11	66	3.6
546	2310	10	4.5	31	84	Trace
415	1749	19	2.6	12	54	7
426	1798	19	2.9	12	56	6.4
432	1816	23	9.2	37	21	3.6
316	1318	9	6	16	44	1.4
210	875	14	2.1	2	19	1.0

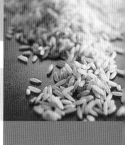

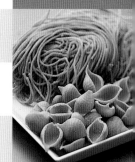

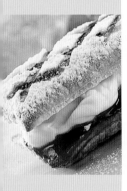

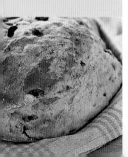

BREAD, CAKES, SCONES AND PASTRIES	AVERAGE PORTION g
Asian pastries	40
Banana loaf, homemade, no icing	85
Battenburg cake	32
Brioche	45
Brown bread, sliced	36
Brown rolls/baps	48
Burfi	40
Carrot cake, homemade, no icing	85
Cheese-topped rolls/baps, white	85
Chelsea buns	78
Cherry cake	38
Chinese flaky pastries	40
Chocolate cake	40
Chocolate cake, with butter icing	65
Chocolate fudge cake	98
Choux buns	112
Ciabatta, plain	50
Coconut cake	40
Cream horns	60
Crispie cakes	31
Croissants	60
Crumpets	40
Currant buns	60
Custard tarts, individual	94
Danish pastries	110
Doughnuts, custard-filled	75
Doughnuts, jam	75
Doughnuts, ring	60
Doughnuts, ring, iced	75
Eccles cake	45
Eclairs, fresh	112
Fancy iced cakes, individual	30
Focaccia, herb/garlic and coriander	50
French baguette, white	40

ENERGY kcal	ENERGY kJ	FAT g	SATURATED FAT g	PROTEIN g	CARBOHYDRATE g	FIBRE g
215	897	16	8	3	17	0.8
230	968	9	5.6	4	35	1.5
118	496	6	1.5	2	16	0.4
144	607	4	2.8	4	24	1.0
75	317	1	0.2	3	15	1.3
113	482	2	0.3	5	22	1.8
117	487	8	4	5	7	0.8
349	1454	25	6.4	5	28	2.1
241	1016	7	3.4	9	38	1.2
285	1203	11	3.3	6	44	1.3
150	630	6	1.6	2	23	0.4
157	659	7	4	2	24	0.8
182	763	11	8.2	3	20	0.5
313	1306	19	14.3	4	33	0.8
351	1479	14	4.5	5	55	0.9
427	1766	36	19	6	20	0.8
135	574	2	0.3	5	26	1.2
174	726	10	2.6	3	20	1
261	1082	21	10	2	15	0.5
144	605	6	3.3	2	23	0.1
224	938	12	5.9	5	26	1.0
83	352	1	0.2	3	18	0.8
178	750	5	2	5	32	1.6
260	1091	14	5.3	6	30	1.1
411	1728	16	6.2	6	56	1.8
269	1125	14	10.4	5	32	1.6
252	1061	11	3.2	4	37	1.6
238	997	13	3.8	4	28	1.4
287	1208	13	3.8	4	41	1.4
214	896	12	4.5	2	27	0.7
418	1746	27	14.3	5	42	0.6
122	515	3	2.8	1	21	0.4
147	620	4	0.6	5	26	0.7
109	465	1	0.1	4	24	1.0

BREAD, CAKES,
SCONES &

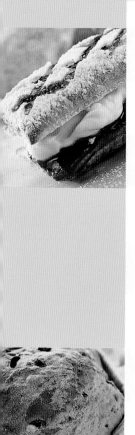

BREAD, CAKES, SCONES AND PASTRIES	AVERAGE PORTION g
French baguette, white, part baked	40
French baton, granary	40
French stick/flute, white	40
Fruit buns, white, not iced	78
Fruit cake, plain	60
Fruit cake, rich	70
Fruit cake, rich, iced	70
Fruit cake, wholemeal	90
Garlic bread	20
Gingerbread	50
Granary bread, sliced	36
Granary rolls	56
Greek pastries	100
Gulab jamen/gulab jambu	40
Hot cross buns	50
Jam tarts	34
Jam tarts, wholemeal	34
Jellabi	40
Madeira	40
Malt loaf, fruit	35
Milk bread, white	15
Mince pies, individual	55
Muffins, English, white	68
Muffins, English, white, toasted	68
Naan bread, garlic and coriander/plain	160
Pitta bread, white	75
Pumpernickel bread	33
Rock cakes	29
Scones, cheese	48
Scones, fruit	48
Scones, plain	48
Scones, potato	57
Scones, wholemeal	50
Scones, wholemeal, fruit	50

ENERGY kcal	ENERGY kJ	FAT g	SATURATED FAT g	PROTEIN g	CARBOHYDRATE g	FIBRE g
108	458	1	0.1	4	23	1.0
110	467	1	0.1	4	22	1.0
101	431	1	0.1	4	21	1.0
218	924	4	1.5	6	41	1.7
212	894	9	3.5	3	35	1.6
239	1007	8	2.4	3	42	1.2
249	1053	8	1.8	3	44	1.2
327	1373	14	4.3	5	48	2.2
73	306	4	1.9	2	9	1.0
190	799	6	1.9	3	32	0.6
87	369	1	0.3	4	18	1.3
133	565	2	0.3	6	24	2.0
322	1349	17	9	5	40	0.8
143	602	6	3	3	21	0.1
155	657	3	1	4	29	0.9
125	527	5	1.6	1	22	0.4
125	528	5	1.6	1	20	1.2
145	611	5	3	2	24	0.5
157	661	6	3.5	2	23	0.4
18	76	1	0.2	3	22.7	0.9
36	153	1	0.2	1	7	0.3
233	975	11	4.1	2	32	1.2
152	644	1	0.3	7	30	1.3
177	753	2	0.3	8	35	1.3
456	1929	12	1.6	12	80	3.2
191	813	1	0.7	7	41	1.8
67	283	1	0.1	2	15	2.1
115	483	5	1	2	18	0.4
174	731	9	4.9	5	21	0.8
152	640	5	1.6	4	25	0.8
174	731	7	2.4	3	26	0.9
169	707	8	4.4	3	22	0.9
163	684	7	2.4	4	22	2.6
162	683	6	2	4	24	2.5

BREAD, CAKES, SCONES & PASTRIES **83**

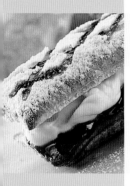

BREAD, CAKES, SCONES AND PASTRIES	AVERAGE PORTION g
Scotch pancakes	31
Slimmers white bread, sliced	20
Soda bread, brown	130
Sponge, fatless	58
Sponge, frozen	60
Sponge, jam-filled	60
Sponge, with butter icing	60
Strawberry tartlets	54
Swiss roll	30
Swiss rolls, chocolate, individual	30
Teacakes	55
Tortilla, soft	160
Vanilla slices	113
Waffles	65
Wheatgerm bread	30
White bread, crusty bloomer	35
White bread, farmhouse, large	35
White bread, farmhouse, small	27
White bread, premium	36
White bread, standard	36
White bread, standard, toasted	36
White rolls, crusty	50
White rolls, soft	45
Wholemeal bread	38
Wholemeal bread, toasted	38
Wholemeal rolls	48

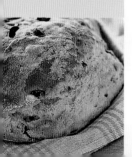

ENERGY kcal	ENERGY kJ	FAT g	SATURATED FAT g	PROTEIN g	CARBOHYDRATE g	FIBRE g
91	381	4	1.3	2	14	0.4
46	193	1	0.1	2	9	0.5
267	1132	4	1.0	11	50	4.9
171	722	4	1	6	31	0.5
190	795	10	3.1	2	24	0.4
181	768	3	1	3	39	1.1
294	1228	18	5.6	3	31	0.4
111	466	6	3.2	1	14	0.6
83	352	1	0.3	2	17	0.2
101	426	5	1.4	1	17	0.3
181	766	5	1.8	5	32	1.2
451	1903	14	2.9	12	73	3.0
373	1563	20	10.6	5	45	0.9
217	911	11	4.7	6	26	1
66	281	1	0.2	3	12	1.2
86	368	1	0.2	3	18	0.8
83	353	1	0.2	3	17	0.7
66	281	1	0.2	2	14	0.7
83	352	1	0.2	3	17	0.7
79	335	1	0.1	3	17	0.7
97	414	1	0.1	3	21	0.0
131	558	1	0.3	5	27	1.2
114	485	1	0.3	4	23	0.9
82	349	1	0.2	4	16	1.9
102	431	1	0.2	5	20	0.0
117	498	2	0.2	5	22	2.1

BREAD, CAKES,
SCONES &

CHEESE

	AVERAGE PORTION g
Brie, without rind	40
Camembert	40
Cheddar, English, white	40
Cheddar, half-fat (15% fat)	40
Cheddar, vegetarian	40
Cheese spread	30
Cheshire, white	40
Cottage (4% fat)	40
Cottage, low-fat (1.5–2% fat)	40
Danish Blue	30
Dolcelatte, without rind	40
Double Gloucester	40
Edam	40
Emmental	40
Fontina	28
Fromage frais, fruit	100
Fromage frais, fruit, virtually fat-free	100
Fromage frais, natural	100
Fromage frais, natural, virtually fat-free	100
Goats' milk	55
Gouda	40
Halloumi	40
Lancashire	40
Mascarpone	55
Monterey Jack	28
Mozzarella, fresh	55
Mozzarella, grated	55
Paneer	40
Parmesan, drums, freshly grated	20
Parmesan, wedges, freshly grated	20
Pecorino	28
Port Salut	40
Processed cheese, slices	20
Provolone	28

Unless otherwise specified, generic cheeses are made with cows' milk.

ENERGY kcal	ENERGY kJ	FAT g	SATURATED FAT g	PROTEIN g	CARBOHYDRATE g	FIBRE g
144	596	12	7.3	8	2	0
116	482	9	6.0	9	Trace	0
166	690	14	8.7	10	0	0
109	456	6	4.3	13	Trace	0
156	647	13	8.3	10	Trace	0
81	335	7	4.7	3	2	0
152	630	13	8.5	9	Trace	0
36	149	2	0.9	5	0	0
28	118	1	0.4	5	0	0
103	425	9	5.7	6	Trace	0
158	652	14	8.7	7	Trace	0
165	684	14	9.3	10	Trace	0
136	566	10	6.3	11	Trace	0
160	663	12	8.2	12	Trace	0
110	462	9	5.4	7	0	0
135	566	5.6	0.0	5.2	16.9	0.4
50	211	0.2	0.0	6.7	5.6	0.4
113	468	8.0	5.6	6.0	4.4	Trace
48	205	0.1	0.0	7.5	4.6	Trace
174	722	14	9.8	12	Trace	0
151	625	12	8.1	10	Trace	0
124	516	9	6.6	10	0	0
153	633	13	8.4	10	Trace	0
230	949	24	16.2	3	Trace	0
107	443	30	5.4	25	0	0
141	587	11	7.6	10	Trace	0
164	680	12	8.1	14	Trace	0
130	539	10	6.2	10	Trace	0
97	403	7	4.6	9	Trace	0
82	343	6	3.9	7	Trace	0
110	459	8	4.8	1	1	0
133	554	10	7.2	10	Trace	0
59	244	5	2.8	4	1	0
99	417	8	4.8	7	1	0

DAIRY
PRODUCTS **87**

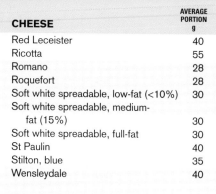

CHEESE	AVERAGE PORTION g
Red Leceister	40
Ricotta	55
Romano	28
Roquefort	28
Soft white spreadable, low-fat (<10%)	30
Soft white spreadable, medium-fat (15%)	30
Soft white spreadable, full-fat	30
St Paulin	40
Stilton, blue	35
Wensleydale	40

CREAM AND SUBSTITUTES	
Cream, clotted	45
Cream, double	30
Cream, half	30
Cream, single	15
Cream, soured	30
Cream, whipping	30
Cream, frozen, whipping	30
Cream, sterilised, canned	45
Cream, UHT, canned spray	10
Cream, UHT, half-fat	15
Cream, UHT, single	15
Cream, UHT, whipping	30
Crème fraîche	50
Crème fraîche, low-fat	50
Mock cream, double	30
Mock cream, single	30
Mock cream, whipping	30

Unless otherwise specified, generic cheeses are made with cows' milk and
cream is fresh.

ENERGY kcal	ENERGY kJ	FAT g	SATURATED FAT g	PROTEIN g	CARBOHYDRATE g	FIBRE g
161	667	13	8.9	10	Trace	0
79	329	6	3.8	5	1	0
110	459	8	4.8	1	1	0
105	438	9	5.4	6	1	0
43	182	2	1.7	4	1	0
56	231	5	3.4	3	Trace	0
94	386	9	6.7	2	Trace	0
133	554	10	7.2	10	Trace	0
143	594	12	8.1	8	Trace	0
152	632	13	8.5	9	Trace	0
264	1086	29	17.9	1	1	0
135	555	16	9	1	1	0
44	184	4	2.5	1	1	0
30	123	3	1.8	0	1	0
62	254	6	3.8	1	1	0
112	462	12	7.4	1	1	0
114	468	12	7.5	1	1	0
108	443	11	6.7	1	2	0
31	127	2	2	0	0	0
21	86	2	1.2	0	1	0
29	122	3	1.8	0	1	0
112	462	12	7.4	1	1	0
190	792	20	13.2	1.2	1.4	0
85	355	7.5	4.5	1.8	2.5	0
136	561	11	8.7	1	1	0
57	236	4	4.2	1	1	0
96	395	9	8.4	1	1	0

EGGS

	AVERAGE PORTION g
Battery, raw	60
Boiled	50
Duck, boiled and salted	70
Duck, raw	75
Egg yolk, raw	18
Free-range, raw	60
Fried in vegetable oil	60
Fried, without fat	50
Poached	50
Quail, raw	40

EGG DISHES

Omelette, cheese	150
Omelette, plain (two-egg)	120
Omelette, Spanish (two-egg)	150
Scrambled, with milk (two-egg)	120
Scrambled, without milk (two-egg)	100

MILK AND MILK SUBSTITUTES

Coffee whitener	3
Condensed milk, skimmed, sweetened	15
Condensed milk, whole, sweetened	15
Evaporated milk, reduced-fat	15
Evaporated milk, whole	15
Flavoured milk	214
Goats' milk, pasteurised	146
Semi-skimmed milk, pasteurised	146
Semi-skimmed milk, UHT	146
Sheep's milk	146
Skimmed milk, dried	3
Skimmed milk, dried, with vegetable fat	3

Unless otherwise specified, figures are for one egg, chicken's eggs are medium-sized and milk is cows' milk.

ENERGY kcal	ENERGY kJ	FAT g	SATURATED FAT g	PROTEIN g	CARBOHYDRATE g	FIBRE g
88	367	1.9	6	8	Trace	0
74	306	1.5	5	6	Trace	0
139	575	2.7	11	10	Trace	0
122	510	2.2	9	11	Trace	0
61	252	1.6	5	3	Trace	0
86	358	1.7	7	7	Trace	0
107	447	2.4	8	8	Trace	0
87	363	1.8	6	8	Trace	0
74	306	1.5	5	6	Trace	0
60	252	1.2	4	5	Trace	0
399	1659	18.3	34	24	Trace	0
229	950	8.9	20	13	Trace	0
180	752	2.4	12	9	9	2.1
296	1230	13.9	27	13	1	0
160	664	3.3	12	14	Trace	0
16	68	1	1	0	2	0
40	171	0	0	2	9	0
50	211	2	0.9	1	8	0
18	77	1	0.2	1	2	0
23	94	1	0.9	1	1	0
146	614	3	1.9	8	23	0
88	369	5	3.4	5	6	0
67	285	2	1.5	5	7	0
67	283	2	1.6	5	7	0
139	578	8	5.5	8	7	0
10	44	0	0	1	2	0
15	61	1	0.5	1	1	0

MILK AND MILK SUBSTITUTES	AVERAGE PORTION g
Skimmed milk, pasteurised	146
Skimmed milk, sterilised	136
Skimmed milk, UHT	146
Soya milk	146
Soya milk, flavoured	146
Whole milk, dried	3
Whole milk, pasteurised	146
Whole milk, sterilised	146
Whole milk, UHT	146

YOGHURTS

Crème fraîche (see under cream)	
Fromage frais (see under cheese)	
Drinking yoghurt	200
Probiotic yoghurt drink, orange	100
Probiotic yoghurt drink, plain	100
Yoghurt, French set, fruit, low-fat	125
Yoghurt, fruit	125
Yoghurt, fruit, low-fat	125
Yoghurt, fruit, virtuallly fat-free	125
Yoghurt, Greek-style, fruit, whole milk	150
Yoghurt, Greek-style, honey, whole milk	150
Yoghurt, Greek-style, natural, whole milk	150
Yoghurt, hazelnut, low-fat	125
Yoghurt, long life, fruit, whole milk	125
Yoghurt, natural, low-fat	125
Yoghurt, natural, virtually fat-free	125
Yoghurt, soya, fruit	125
Yoghurt, toffee, low-fat	125
Yoghurt, twin pot, fruit, virtually fat-free	135
Yoghurt, vanilla, low-fat	125

Unless otherwise specified, milk is cows' milk.

ENERGY kcal	ENERGY kJ	FAT g	SATURATED FAT g	PROTEIN g	CARBOHYDRATE g	FIBRE g
48	204	1	0.1	5	7	0
44	188	1	0.1	5	7	0
47	200	1	0.1	5	7	0
47	193	2	0.4	4	1	Trace
58	245	2	0.3	4	5	Trace
15	62	1	0.5	1	1	0
96	402	6	3.5	5	7	0
96	404	6	3.5	5	7	0
96	402	6	3.5	5	7	0
124	526	Trace	Trace	6	26	Trace
67	279	0.9	0.6	1.5	13.4	1.3
68	284	1	0.7	1.7	13.1	1.4
103	435	1.4	1.0	4.3	19.5	0.3
133	564	3.8	2.5	4.9	21.4	0.3
97	412	1.4	0.9	5.1	17.1	0.3
75	318	0.5	0.0	5.9	12.5	0.3
205	857	12.6	8.4	7.2	16.8	Trace
221	927	12.5	8.4	7.7	21.0	Trace
198	824	15.3	10.2	8.4	7.2	Trace
111	469	1.9	0.8	5.5	19.1	0.3
125	529	4.3	0.0	3.9	19.1	0.3
69	294	1.3	0.9	5.9	9.3	Trace
67	286	0.3	0.0	6.6	10.3	Trace
92	388	2.3	0.3	2.9	16.0	0.4
114	484	1.1	0.8	4.8	22.6	Trace
55	236	0.1	0.1	4.5	9.7	0.7
114	484	1.1	0.8	4.8	22.6	Trace

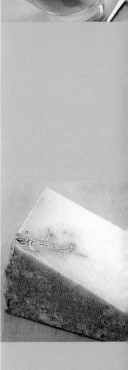

FATS	AVERAGE PORTION g
Butter	
Butter	20
Ghee	7
Margarine	
Hard, animal and vegetable fats	10
Hard, vegetable fats	10
Soft, animal and vegetable fat	7
Soft, polyunsaturated	7
Other fats	
Compound cooking fat	15
Compound cooking fat, polyunsaturated	15
Dripping, beef	15
Ghee, vegetable	7
Lard	15
Suet, beef, shredded	15
Suet, vegetable	15
Spreads	
Blended 70% fat	7
Blended 40% fat	7
20–25% fat, not polyunsaturated	7
20–25% fat	7
35–40% fat	7
40% fat, not polyunsaturated	7
5% fat	7
60% fat	7
60% fat, with olive oil	7
70% fat	7

OILS	
Corn oil	15
Grapeseed oil	11
Hazelnut oil	2

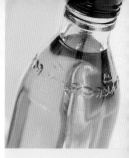

ENERGY kcal	ENERGY kJ	FAT g	SATURATED FAT g	PROTEIN g	CARBOHYDRATE g	FIBRE g
147	606	16	11	0	Trace	0
63	259	7	4.6	Trace	Trace	0
72	295	8	3.5	0	0	0
74	304	8	3.6	0	0	0
52	213	6	1.9	0	0	0
52	215	6	1.2	Trace	0	0
135	554	15	7.4	Trace	0	0
135	554	15	3.1	Trace	Trace	0
134	549	15	7.9	Trace	Trace	0
63	257	7	3.4	Trace	Trace	0
134	549	15	6	Trace	0	0
124	510	14	7.5	Trace	2	0.1
125	517	13	6.8	0	2	0
48	196	5	1.8	0	0	0
27	113	3	1.3	0	0	0
17	71	2	0.4	0	0	0
13	53	1	0.3	0	0	0
26	105	3	0.6	0	0	0
28	113	3	0.8	0	0	0
7	30	1	0.1	0	1	0.4
39	159	4	0.8	0	0	0
40	164	4	0.8	0	0	0
44	183	5	0.9	0	0	0
135	554	15	2.2	Trace	0	0
99	407	11	1.2	Trace	0	0
99	407	11	0.9	Trace	0	0

OILS	AVERAGE PORTION g
Olive oil	11
Palm oil	11
Peanut oil	11
Rapeseed oil	11
Safflower oil	11
Sesame oil	3
Soya oil	11
Sunflower oil	11
Vegetable oil	11
Walnut oil	11
Wheatgerm oil	11

ENERGY kcal	ENERGY kJ	FAT g	SATURATED FAT g	PROTEIN g	CARBOHYDRATE g	FIBRE g
99	407	11	1.6	Trace	0	0
99	407	11	5.3	Trace	0	0
99	407	11	2.2	Trace	0	0
99	407	11	0.7	Trace	0	0
99	407	11	1.1	Trace	0	0
27	111	3	0.4	Trace	0	0
99	407	11	1.7	Trace	0	0
99	407	11	1.3	Trace	0	0
99	407	11	1.1	Trace	0	0
99	407	11	1	Trace	0	0
99	407	11	2	Trace	0	0

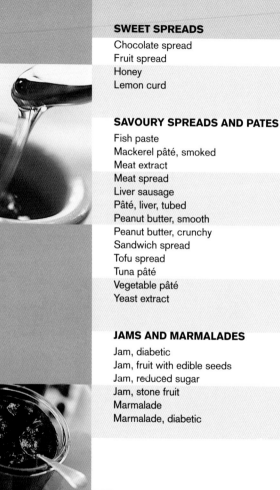

SWEET SPREADS	AVERAGE PORTION g
Chocolate spread	16
Fruit spread	16
Honey	17
Lemon curd	15

SAVOURY SPREADS AND PATES

Fish paste	10
Mackerel pâté, smoked	40
Meat extract	9
Meat spread	10
Liver sausage	40
Pâté, liver, tubed	40
Peanut butter, smooth	25
Peanut butter, crunchy	25
Sandwich spread	15
Tofu spread	45
Tuna pâté	40
Vegetable pâté	80
Yeast extract	9

JAMS AND MARMALADES

Jam, diabetic	15
Jam, fruit with edible seeds	15
Jam, reduced sugar	15
Jam, stone fruit	15
Marmalade	15
Marmalade, diabetic	15

Unless otherwise specified, spreads are made with polyunsaturated fats.

ENERGY kcal	ENERGY kJ	FAT g	SATURATED FAT g	PROTEIN g	CARBOHYDRATE g	FIBRE g
91	380	6	0.9	1	9	0.2
19	83	Trace	Trace	0	5	0.1
49	209	0	0	0	13	0
42	180	1	0.2	0	9	0
17	71	1	0.5	2	0	0
147	608	14	2.5	5	1	Trace
16	68	0	0	4	0	0
19	80	1	0.6	2	0	Trace
90	377	7	2.1	5	2	0.3
114	472	10	3	5	0	Trace
156	645	13	2.9	6	3	1.4
152	628	13	2.4	6	2	1.5
28	117	1	0.2	0	4	0.1
94	349	9	1.3	2	1	0.2
94	393	7	3.1	7	0	Trace
138	574	11	6	6	5	2
16	69	0	0	4	0	0
26	109	0	0	0	9	0.1
39	167	0	0	0	10	0.1
18	78	Trace	Trace	0	5	0.1
39	167	0	0	0	10	0.1
39	167	0	0	0	10	0
26	109	0	0	0	9	0.1

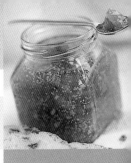

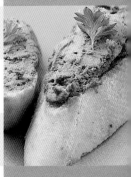

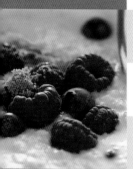

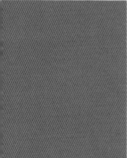

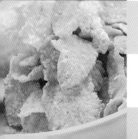

BREAKFAST CEREALS	AVERAGE PORTION g
Bran, flakes	30
Bran, flakes with oat	30
Bran, strands	40
Bran, sultana	30
Bran, with oat and wheat	50
Corn flakes	30
Corn flakes, with nuts	30
Crunchy clusters with fruit	50
Crunchy clusters with chocolate	50
Frosted flakes	30
Fruit and fibre breakfast cereal	40
Hoops, honey	30
Hoops, honey and nut	30
Malted flakes	30
Muesli	50
Muesli, Swiss-style	50
Muesli, with extra fruit	50
Muesli, with no added sugar	50
Multigrain flakes	30
Oat cereal with fruit and nuts	50
Oat cereal with tropical fruit	50
Oat clusters	30
Oat flakes	30
Porridge, instant, made with water	180
Porridge, made with milk and water	160
Porridge, made with water	160
Porridge, made with whole milk	160
Puffed wheat	20
Rice pops	30
Rice pops, chocolate	30
Wheat, shredded	45
Wheat, shredded, honey and nut	40
Wheat, shredded, mini	45
Wholewheat biscuits	20

All values are without any sugar added.

ENERGY kcal	ENERGY kJ	FAT g	SATURATED FAT g	PROTEIN g	CARBOHYDRATE g	FIBRE g
95	406	1	0.1	3	21	3.9
105	435	2	0.2	3	20	3
104	444	1	0.2	6	19	9.8
96	405	1	0.1	3	18	3.9
163	691	2	0.3	5	34	8.9
108	461	Trace	0	2	26	0.3
119	507	1	0.2	2	27	0.2
139	580	5	1.7	4	20	1.3
220	917	8	2.7	3	33	2.4
113	482	Trace	0	2	28	0.2
147	614	2	1.2	2	28	2.2
111	465	1	0.2	2	23	2.1
112	474	1	0.3	2	23	1.5
186	773	1	0.1	3	23	1.3
184	770	3	0.7	6	33	3.2
182	770	3	0.4	5	36	3.2
186	789	3	0.4	5	37	3.2
183	776	4	0.8	5	34	3.8
111	465	Trace	Trace	5	22	0.7
213	888	8	3	5	31	2
217	905	7	4	4	34	3
116	490	3	0.8	3	20	2.7
107	456	1	0.2	3	22	3
671	2844	14	2.2	21	123	13
133	557	5	2.3	5	18	1.3
78	334	2	0.3	2	14	1.3
186	781	8	4.3	8	22	1.3
64	273	Trace	0	3	13	1.1
111	472	0.1	0.1	2	27	0.2
115	491	0.1	0.1	2	28	0.2
150	630	1	0.2	5	30	5.2
152	642	3	0.9	4	28	4.1
154	655	1	0.2	4	32	5
70	300	0.1	0.1	2	15	1.9

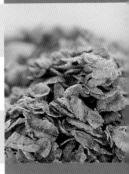

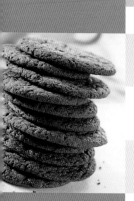

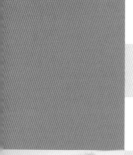

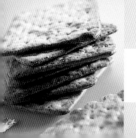

	AVERAGE PORTION g
SAVOURY BISCUITS	
Cheese sandwiches	24
Cream crackers	14
Oatcakes, shop bought	26
Water biscuits	16
Wholemeal crackers	20
CRISPBREADS	
Breadsticks (4)	28
Crispbakes	16
Crispbread, rye	20
French toast	16
Matzos	20
Melba toast	6
Rice cakes	16
SWEET BISCUITS	
All-butter biscuits	19
Bourbon creams	28
Brandy snaps	30
Chocolate, full-coated	50
Chocolate-covered teacakes	26
Coconut biscuits	40
Cookies, chocolate chip	22
Cookies, chocolate chip and hazelnut (1)	24
Cookies, Danish butter	22
Cookies, stem ginger	32
Crunch biscuits	27
Custard creams	24
Custard creams, reduced fat	24
Digestives, chocolate, half coated	26
Digestives, milk chocolate, reduced fat	34

Unless otherwise specified, a helping is two biscuits.

ENERGY kcal	ENERGY kJ	FAT g	SATURATED FAT g	PROTEIN g	CARBOHYDRATE g	FIBRE g
123	516	5	3.5	1	17	0.2
62	260	2	0.4	1	10	0.3
115	482	4	1	3	16	1.3
70	297	1	Trace	2	12	0.5
83	349	2	1	2	14	0.9
108	464	4	1.6	4	20	0.8
60	250	Trace	Trace	2	12	0.6
64	273	0.1	0.1	2	14	2.3
63	262	1	0.5	2	12	0.5
77	327	0	0	2	17	0.6
23	94	Trace	Trace	1	4	0.3
56	234	Trace	Trace	2	12	0.8
90	378	4	3.4	Trace	14	0.2
136	566	6	3.6	2	20	0.6
131	550	6	3	1	19	0.2
262	1099	13	8.4	3	34	1
116	438	4	2.2	2	16	0.4
202	846	12	6	2	21	2
112	461	6	2.7	1	14	0.4
120	504	6	2.6	2	14	0.4
112	461	5	4	1	14	0.3
157	653	9	1.9	1	20	0.6
135	562	7	3.5	2	17	0.6
122	508	6	3.6	2	16	0.4
114	472	4	2.6	2	18	0.4
128	538	6	3.2	2	17	0.6
158	660	10	6	2	24	0.6

SWEET BISCUITS	AVERAGE PORTION g
Digestives, plain	26
Digestives, reduced fat	28
Flapjacks (1 piece)	70
Gingernuts	20
Jaffa cakes	26
Jam rings	38
Jam sandwich creams	30
Malted milk	16
Malted milk creams	26
Marshmallow teacakes, chocolate-coated	28
Morning coffee	10
Nice	20
Nice creams	28
Rich tea	14
Shortbread	26
Shortbread, chocolate chip	40
Shortbread, reduced sugar (1)	33
Snowballs	42
Wafers, filled	14

Unless otherwise specified, a helping is two biscuits.

ENERGY kcal	ENERGY kJ	FAT g	SATURATED FAT g	PROTEIN g	CARBOHYDRATE g	FIBRE g
122	514	5	2.2	2	18	0.6
130	542	6	2	2	20	1
339	1420	19	5.3	3	42	1.9
91	385	3	1.4	1	16	0.3
94	398	3	0.6	1	18	0.4
171	715	6	2.7	2	27	0.6
142	592	6	3.2	2	20	0.6
78	324	3	1.8	1	11	0.3
130	542	6	3.7	2	17	0.4
126	525	5	3	1	18	0.4
45	188	1	0.6	1	7	0.2
94	393	4	2.3	1	12	0.3
140	584	6	3.2	2	18	0.6
64	270	2	1.1	1	10	0.2
129	543	7	4.5	2	17	0.5
206	858	10	8.6	2	24	0.6
156	652	9	5.9	2	18	0.5
196	814	10	9.8	2	24	2.2
75	314	4	2.6	1	9	0.3

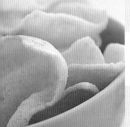

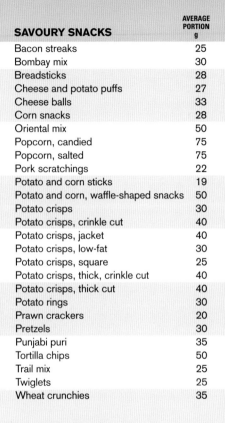

SAVOURY SNACKS	AVERAGE PORTION g
Bacon streaks	25
Bombay mix	30
Breadsticks	28
Cheese and potato puffs	27
Cheese balls	33
Corn snacks	28
Oriental mix	50
Popcorn, candied	75
Popcorn, salted	75
Pork scratchings	22
Potato and corn sticks	19
Potato and corn, waffle-shaped snacks	50
Potato crisps	30
Potato crisps, crinkle cut	40
Potato crisps, jacket	40
Potato crisps, low-fat	30
Potato crisps, square	25
Potato crisps, thick, crinkle cut	40
Potato crisps, thick cut	40
Potato rings	30
Prawn crackers	20
Pretzels	30
Punjabi puri	35
Tortilla chips	50
Trail mix	25
Twiglets	25
Wheat crunchies	35

ENERGY kcal	ENERGY kJ	FAT g	SATURATED FAT g	PROTEIN g	CARBOHYDRATE g	FIBRE g
113	473	5	1.6	2	16	0.5
151	630	10	1.2	6	11	1.9
108	464	4	1.6	4	20	0.8
140	585	9	3.2	2	15	0.3
148	621	8	1.8	2	19	0.8
141	591	9	3.8	1	16	1
273	1142	20	3	10	17	0.3
360	1514	14	1.5	2	58	1
445	1851	32	3.2	5	37	1
133	554	10	3.6	11	0	0.1
88	368	4	1.3	1	11	0.6
241	1009	12	2.8	2	32	1.3
159	665	10	4.2	2	16	1.6
219	913	14	5.8	2	22	2.3
204	851	13	5.3	3	21	1.9
137	577	6	2.8	2	19	1.8
108	454	5	2.2	2	14	1.1
203	848	12	5	2	22	1.6
200	836	11	4.6	3	23	1.6
157	656	10	4.2	1	18	0.8
103	432	7	1.9	0	11	0.3
114	479	1	0.2	3	24	0.8
188	784	12	2.9	3	18	0.9
230	964	11	2	4	30	3
108	451	7	1.3	2	9	1.1
96	404	3	1.2	3	16	2.6
158	662	7	3.2	4	21	1.2

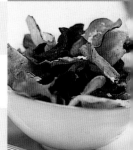

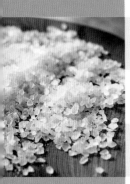

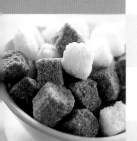

FLOUR	AVERAGE PORTION g
Chapati, brown	100
Chapati, white	100
Cornflour	30
Rye, whole	20
Wheat, brown	100
Wheat, white, breadmaking	100
Wheat, white, plain	100
Wheat, white, self-raising	100
Wheat, wholemeal	100

GRAVY AND STOCK CUBES	
Instant granules	5
Instant granules, made up	45
Stock cubes, beef/chicken	7
Stock cubes, vegetable	7

BAKING INGREDIENTS	
Baking powder	4
Marzipan, shop bought	25
Mincemeat	28
Mincemeat, vegetarian	28
Yeast, bakers', compressed	5
Yeast, dried	5

MISCELLANEOUS	
Bran, wheat	7
Coconut, creamed block	25
Coconut, desiccated	28
Custard powder	30
Gelatine	3
Olives, in brine, stoned	18

ENERGY kcal	ENERGY kJ	FAT g	SATURATED FAT g	PROTEIN g	CARBOHYDRATE g	FIBRE g
333	1419	1	0.2	12	74	6
335	1426	1	0.1	10	78	3
106	452	0	0	0	28	0
67	286	1	0.1	2	15	2.3
323	1377	2	0.2	13	69	6.4
341	1451	1	0.2	12	75	3.1
341	1450	1	0.2	9	78	3.1
330	1407	1	0.2	9	76	3.1
310	1318	2	0.3	13	64	9
23	96	2	Trace	0	2	Trace
15	64	1	Trace	0	1	Trace
17	69	1	Trace	1	1	0
18	74	1	Trace	1	1	Trace
7	28	0	0	0	2	0
101	426	3	0.3	1	17	0.5
77	326	1	Trace	0	17	0.4
85	359	4	Trace	0	12	0.4
3	11	0	0	1	0	Trace
8	36	0	0	2	0	Trace
14	61	1	0.1	1	2	2.5
167	690	17	14.8	2	2	2
169	698	17	15	2	2	3.8
106	452	0	0	0	28	0
10	43	0	0	3	0	0
19	76	2	0.3	0	Trace	0.5

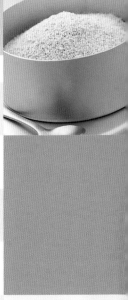

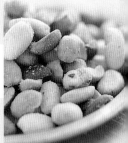

STORECUPBOARD INGREDIENTS

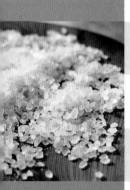

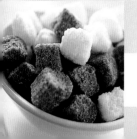

MISCELLANEOUS	AVERAGE PORTION g
Salt	5
Tomatoes, sundried, bottled in oil	10
Vinegar	15
Wheatgerm	5

PURÉES	
Tomato purée	20
Vegetable purée	20

SUGARS, SYRUPS AND TREACLE	
Jaggery	16
Sugar, brown	20
Sugar, Demerara	20
Sugar, icing	20
Sugar, white	20
Syrup, golden	55
Syrup, golden, pouring	50
Syrup, maple	55
Treacle, black	50

NUTS AND SEEDS	
Almonds, toasted	13
Barcelona nuts	15
Brazil nuts	10
Cashew nuts, plain	10
Cashew nuts, roasted and salted	25
Chestnuts	50
Coconut, fresh	28
Hazelnuts	10
Macadamia nuts, salted	10
Melon seeds	15

ENERGY kcal	ENERGY kJ	FAT g	SATURATED FAT g	PROTEIN g	CARBOHYDRATE g	FIBRE g
0	0	0	0	0	0	0
50	204	5	0.7	0	1	0.5
3	13	0	0	0	0	0
18	75	0	0.1	1	2	0.8
15	65	Trace	Trace	1	3	0.6
14	51	1	0	1	1	0.6
59	250	0	0	0	16	0
72	309	0	0	0	20	0
79	336	0	0	0	21	0
79	336	0	0	Trace	21	0
79	336	0	0	Trace	21	0
164	698	0	0	0	43	0
148	632	0	0	Trace	40	0
144	602	Trace	Trace	0	37	0
129	548	0	0	1	34	Trace
81	334	7	0.6	3	1	1
96	396	10	2.3	2	1	1
68	281	7	1.6	1	0	0.4
57	237	5	1	2	2	0.3
153	633	13	2.5	5	5	0.8
85	360	1	0.3	1	18	2
98	405	10	8.7	1	1	2
65	269	6	0.5	1	1	0.7
75	308	8	1.1	1	0	0.5
87	363	7	1.8	4	1	0.8

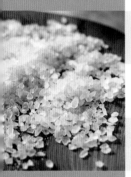

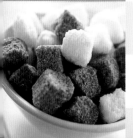

NUTS AND SEEDS	AVERAGE PORTION g
Mixed nuts	40
Mixed nuts and raisins	40
Peanuts, dry roasted	40
Peanuts, plain	13
Peanuts, roasted and salted	25
Pecan nuts	60
Pine nuts	5
Pistachio nuts, roasted and salted	10
Pumpkin seeds	16
Sesame seeds	12
Sunflower seeds	16
Walnuts	20

ENERGY kcal	ENERGY kJ	FAT g	SATURATED FAT g	PROTEIN g	CARBOHYDRATE g	FIBRE g
243	1006	22	3.4	9	3	2.4
192	802	14	2.2	6	13	1.8
236	976	20	3.6	10	4	2.6
73	304	6	1.1	3	2	0.8
151	623	13	2.4	6	2	1.5
413	1706	42	3.4	6	3	2.8
34	142	3	0.2	1	0	0.1
60	249	6	0.7	2	1	0.6
91	378	7	1.1	4	2	0.8
72	296	7	1	2	0	0.9
96	400	8	0.8	3	3	1
138	567	14	1.1	3	1	0.7

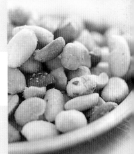

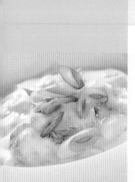

TABLE SAUCES	**AVERAGE PORTION g**
Apple sauce, homemade	20
Brown sauce	20
Brown sauce, hot	20
Brown sauce, sweet	20
Chilli sauce	25
Horseradish sauce	20
Mint sauce	10
Mustard, powder, made up	8
Mustard, smooth	2
Mustard, wholegrain	14
Soy sauce, dark, thick	5
Soy sauce, light, thin	5
Tartare sauce	30
Tomato ketchup	20

WHITE SAUCES	
Bread sauce, made with semi-skimmed milk	45
Bread sauce, made with whole milk	45
Cheese sauce, made with semi-skimmed milk	62
Cheese sauce, made with whole milk	62
Onion sauce, made with semi-skimmed milk	62
Onion sauce, made with whole milk	62
White sauce, savoury, made with semi-skimmed milk	62
White sauce, savoury, made with whole milk	62
White sauce, sweet, made with semi-skimmed milk	62
White sauce, sweet, made with whole milk	62

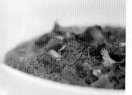

ENERGY kcal	ENERGY kJ	FAT g	SATURATED FAT g	PROTEIN g	CARBOHYDRATE g	FIBRE g
13	55	0	0	0	3	0.2
20	84	Trace	Trace	0	5	0.1
24	102	Trace	Trace	0	6	0.1
20	84	Trace	Trace	0	4	0.1
20	84	Trace	Trace	0	4	0.3
31	128	2	0.2	1	4	0.5
10	43	Trace	Trace	0	2	0.2
18	75	1	0.1	1	0	0
3	12	0	0	0	0	0
20	82	1	0.1	1	5	Trace
3	13	0	0	0	6	0.2
3	13	Trace	Trace	0	1	0.7
90	372	7	0.5	0	0	0.2
23	98	Trace	Trace	0	1	0.7
42	177	1	0.6	2	6	0.1
50	208	2	1.2	2	6	0.1
112	465	8	3.9	4	6	0.1
122	508	8	4.8	4	6	0.1
53	224	3	1.1	2	5	0.2
61	257	4	1.7	2	5	0.2
79	334	5	1.8	3	7	0.1
93	387	6	2.7	3	7	0.1
93	393	4	1.7	2	12	0.1
105	441	6	2.5	2	12	0.1

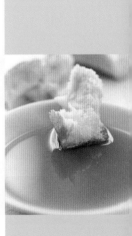

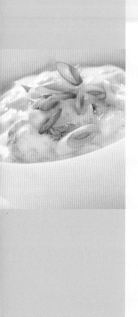

	AVERAGE PORTION g
CHUTNEYS	
Chutney, apple, homemade	33
Chutney, mango, oily	33
Chutney, mango, sweet	33
Chutney, mixed fruit	33
Chutney, tomato	33
DIPS	
Dips, sour-cream-based	30
Guacamole	45
Hummus	30
Taramasalata	45
Tzatziki	45
DRESSINGS	
Blue cheese	25
'Fat-free'	15
French	15
Low-fat	15
Oil and lemon	15
Thousand island	30
Thousand island, reduced-calorie	30
Yogurt-based	30
MAYONNAISE AND SALAD CREAM	
Mayonnaise	30
Mayonnaise, homemade, made with lemon juice	30
Mayonnaise, homemade, made with vinegar	30
Mayonnaise, reduced-calorie	30

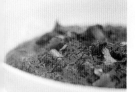

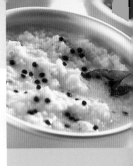

ENERGY kcal	ENERGY kJ	FAT g	SATURATED FAT g	PROTEIN g	CARBOHYDRATE g	FIBRE g
66	283	Trace	Trace	0	17	0.4
94	397	4	Trace	0	16	0.3
62	266	Trace	Trace	0	16	0.3
51	219	Trace	Trace	0	13	0.3
42	179	Trace	Trace	0	10	0.4
108	445	11	3.7	1	1	Trace
58	239	6	1.2	1	1	1.1
56	234	4	0.5	2	3	0.7
227	935	24	1.8	1	2	Trace
30	124	2	1.3	2	1	0.1
114	472	12	6.2	1	2	0
10	42	0	0	0	2	0
69	285	7	0.6	0	1	0
11	45	1	0.1	0	1	Trace
97	399	11	1.1	0	0	Trace
97	401	9	0.9	0	4	0.1
59	243	5	0.5	0	4	Trace
88	363	8	0.8	1	3	Trace
207	853	23	3.3	0	1	0
237	974	26	3.8	1	0	Trace
217	894	24	3.5	1	0	0
86	356	8	1.1	0	2	0

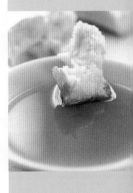

MAYONNAISE AND SALAD CREAM	AVERAGE PORTION g
Salad cream	20
Salad cream, reduced-calorie	20

PICKLES	
Gherkins, pickled	25
Onions, pickled	30
Piccalilli	40
Pickle, chilli, oily	15
Pickle, chow chow, sour	15
Pickle, chow chow, sweet	15
Pickle, lime, oily	15
Pickle, mango, oily	15
Pickle, mixed vegetables	15
Pickle, sweet	15

COOKING SAUCES	
Barbecue sauce	25
Black bean sauce	20
Chilli sauce	25
Cook-in-sauces, canned, different flavours	150
Curry sauce, canned	150
Oyster sauce	15
Sauce, curry, sweet	150
Sauce, curry, tomato and onion	150
Soy sauce, dark, thick	5
Soy sauce, light, thin	5
Tomato sauce	90
Pasta sauce, tomato based	170

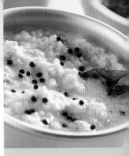

ENERGY kcal	ENERGY kJ	FAT g	SATURATED FAT g	PROTEIN g	CARBOHYDRATE g	FIBRE g
70	288	6	0.8	0	3	0
39	161	3	0.5	0	2	0
4	15	Trace	Trace	0	1	0.3
7	30	Trace	Trace	0	1	0.4
34	144	0	0	0	7	0.4
41	168	4	Trace	0	1	0.2
4	18	0	0	0	1	0.2
17	73	0	0	0	4	0.2
27	111	2	Trace	0	1	0.2
27	110	2	Trace	0	1	0.2
3	14	0	0	0	1	0.2
21	91	0	Trace	0	5	0.2
23	99	0	0	0	6	0.1
19	79	0	0	1	2	0.4
20	84	Trace	Trace	0	4	0.3
65	272	4	0.2	2	12	Trace
117	486	8	0.4	2	11	Trace
12	51	0	Trace	1	3	Trace
137	570	8	2.3	2	14	2.1
297	1229	29	3	3	9	1.7
3	13	0	0	0	0	00
3	13	0	0	0	0	0
80	337	5	1.6	2	8	1.3
80	340	3	0.3	3	12	2.5

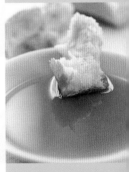

CUSTARDS

	AVERAGE PORTION g
Crème caramel	90
Custard, canned, ready-to-serve	120
Custard, canned, ready-to-serve, low-fat	120
Custard, chilled, ready-to-serve	120
Custard, confectioners'	150
Custard, made with semi-skimmed milk	150
Custard, made with whole milk	120

ENERGY kcal	ENERGY kJ	FAT g	SATURATED FAT g	PROTEIN g	CARBOHYDRATE g	FIBRE g
98	416	1	Trace	3	19	Trace
118	497	3	2.3	3	20	0.0
93	395	2	0.0	3	18	0.0
135	569	6	4.4	3	18	0.0
255	1077	9	4.1	10	37	0.3
141	605	3	1.8	6	25	Trace
140	594	5	3.4	4	20	Trace

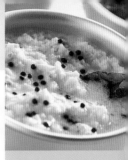

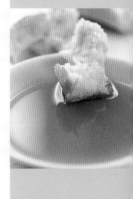

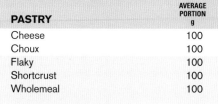

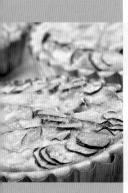

PASTRY	AVERAGE PORTION g
Cheese	100
Choux	100
Flaky	100
Shortcrust	100
Wholemeal	100

PASTRY DISHES	
Beef pie, shop bought	141
Chicken and mushroom pie, single crust	100
Chicken pie, individual, baked	130
Cornish pasty	155
Cornish pasty, shop bought	155
Lamb samosa, baked	70
Lamb samosa, deep-fried	70
Pasty, vegetable	155
Pasty, vegetable, wholemeal	155
Pork and egg pie	60
Pork pie	60
Pork pie, mini	50
Quiche, broccoli	140
Quiche, broccoli, wholemeal	140
Quiche, cauliflower cheese	140
Quiche, cauliflower cheese, wholemeal	140
Quiche, cheese and egg	140
Quiche, cheese and egg, wholemeal	140
Quiche, cheese and mushroom	140
Quiche, cheese and mushroom, wholemeal	140
Quiche, cheese, onion and potato	140
Quiche, cheese, onion and potato, wholemeal	140
Quiche, mushroom	140

Unless otherwise specified, all pastry dishes are homemade.

ENERGY kcal	ENERGY kJ	FAT g	SATURATED FAT g	PROTEIN g	CARBOHYDRATE g	FIBRE g
500	2083	34	15.3	13	37	1.5
325	1355	20	15	9	30	1.2
560	2332	41	14.7	6	46	1.8
521	2174	32	11.7	7	54	2.2
499	2080	33	11.8	9	45	6.3
437	1826	24	11.8	12	38	0.7
200	836	10	4.5	13	14	0.6
374	1563	21	9.1	12	32	1
456	1905	28	9.8	10	43	2.6
414	1731	25	9.1	10	39	1.4
187	781	10	2.5	8	16	1.2
265	1097	22	3.3	6	12	0.8
425	1783	23	5.7	6	52	2.9
406	1702	24	5.7	8	43	6.4
178	740	13	4.4	6	10	0.5
228	947	18	6.8	6	11	0.5
196	815	14	5.7	5	13	0.5
349	1455	21	8.3	12	30	1.7
337	1408	21	8.3	13	25	3.8
277	1156	18	7.1	7	24	1.5
269	1121	18	7.1	8	20	3.1
440	1834	31	14.4	18	24	0.8
431	1796	31	14.6	18	20	2.7
396	1655	26	10.8	15	26	1.3
388	1616	27	10.8	16	22	3.1
480	2005	33	16	18	28	1.4
472	1966	34	16.1	19	25	3.1
398	1659	27	12.2	14	26	1.3

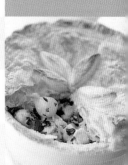

PASTRY DISHES

	AVERAGE PORTION g
Quiche, mushroom, wholemeal	140
Quiche, spinach	140
Quiche, spinach, wholemeal	140
Quiche, vegetable	140
Quiche, vegetable, wholemeal	140
Sausage rolls, flaky pastry	60
Sausage rolls, shortcrust pastry	60
Steak and kidney pie, double crust	120
Steak and kidney pie, shop bought	141

Unless otherwise specified, all pastry dishes are homemade.

ENERGY kcal	ENERGY kJ	FAT g	SATURATED FAT g	PROTEIN g	CARBOHYDRATE g	FIBRE g
388	1618	28	12.2	15	21	3.1
287	1203	18	5.6	14	18	2
281	1176	18	5.6	15	16	3.2
295	1238	18	6	7	28	2.1
286	1197	18	6	8	24	3.9
238	991	17	6.5	6	15	0.8
229	953	16	5.8	6	17	0.9
406	1694	26	9.7	16	27	1.1
437	1826	24	11.8	12	38	0.7

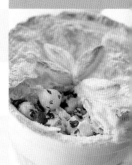

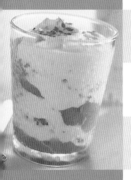

MILK-BASED PUDDINGS AND DESSERTS	AVERAGE PORTION g
Blancmange	150
Fruit fool	120
Fruit fool, low-fat	120
Milk pudding, made with semi-skimmed milk	200
Milk pudding, made with whole milk	200
Rice desserts, individual, with fruit	135
Rice pudding, canned	200
Tiramisu	90
Trifle, chocolate	113
Trifle, fruit	113

CHEESECAKES	
Chocolate	120
Frozen	90
Fruit, individual	90
Fruit, large	120

OTHER DESSERTS	
Christmas pudding	100
Crumble, fruit	170
Jelly, made with water	115
Pavlova, chocolate	100
Pavlova, fruit	100
Profiteroles with chocolate sauce	155
Strudel, fruit	115

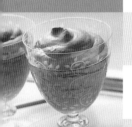

MOUSSE	
Chocolate, individual	60
Chocolate	60
Fruit	60

ENERGY kcal	ENERGY kJ	FAT g	SATURATED FAT g	PROTEIN g	CARBOHYDRATE g	FIBRE g
171	720	6	3.4	5	27	Trace
213	890	13	8.8	3	22	0.5
97	405	6	0.0	4	8	0.5l
214	914	4	2.2	8	40	0.2
258	1086	9	5.4	8	40	0.2
153	648	3	2.0	4	29	0.4
178	748	3	3.2	7	28	0.4
220	919	13	7.7	4	24	0.4
233	971	17	10.7	5	15	1.4
161	672	10	6.3	3	15	2.4
415	1731	28	14.4	6	37	0.8
218	915	10	5	5	30	0.8
238	1000	11	6.8	5	31	0.9
353	1477	19	11.8	5	42	1.0
291	1227	10	4.5	5	50	1.3
373	1571	14	6.7	4	61	2.2
70	299	0	0	1	17	0
370	1552	20	10.7	4	47	0.3
288	1210	13	7.1	3	42	0.3
535	2226	40	21.7	9	38	1.1
279	1167	16	6.0	3	33	1.2
83	352	4	2.7	2	12	0.1
73	310	2	1.5	3	11	0.1
82	345	3	2	3	11	0.1

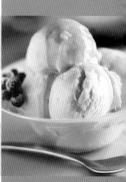

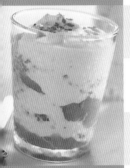

PIES

	AVERAGE PORTION g
Apple pie, deep filled, double crust	110
Apple pie, double crust	110
Banoffee pie	150
Lemon meringue pie	150
Mince pies, individual	55
Mississippi mud pie	150

ICE CREAM AND FROZEN DESSERTS

Arctic roll	50
Banana split	100
Chocolate-covered ice cream bar	51
Chocolate nut sundae	60
Frozen ice cream dessert, chocolate	60
Frozen ice cream dessert, plain	60
Ice cream, chocolate	75
Ice cream, dairy-free	75
Ice cream, fruit	75
Ice cream, luxury, vanilla	75
Ice cream, soya	75
Ice cream, vanilla	75
Ice cream, virtually fat free	75
Ice cream bar, chocolate flavoured coating	48
Ice cream cone, chocolate/mint/nuts	73
Ice cream cone, strawberry	81
Knickerbocker glory	100
Kulfi	80
Lolly, fruit	73
Lolly, ice cream, with fruit coating	73
Peach melba	60
Sorbet, fruit	75

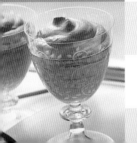

ENERGY kcal	ENERGY kJ	FAT g	SATURATED FAT g	PROTEIN g	CARBOHYDRATE g	FIBRE g
281	1183	12	3.8	4	42	1.1
269	1129	14	4.5	4	33	1.1
478	1997	30	15.0	6	49	3.8
377	1590	13	4.6	4	65	0.7
233	975	11	4.1	2	32	1.2
478	1997	30	15.0	6	49	3.8
100	424	3	1.5	2	17	Trace
182	761	11	6	2	19	0.6
163	679	2	7.7	3	12	0
167	699	9	5	2	21	0.1
150	627	11	8.5	2	13	0.0
136	568	9	6.7	2	14	Trace
156	653	8	5.2	3	19	0.0
156	654	9	2.8	2	17	0.1
119	499	5	3.4	2	17	0.2
161	670	11	6.8	3	13	0.0
156	654	9	2.8	2	17	0.1
115	480	6	3.6	2	14	0.0
76	324	1	Trace	3	15	0.0
142	590	10	8.8	2	11	0.0
207	867	13	9.6	3	21	0.2
201	844	10	7.1	3	28	0.2
112	473	5	2.9	2	16	0.2
339	1405	32	18.2	4	9	0.5
56	234	1	0.1	0	14	0.1
78	326	2	1	1	15	0.1
98	411	6	3.8	1	10	0.2
98	422	Trace	Trace	1	26	0

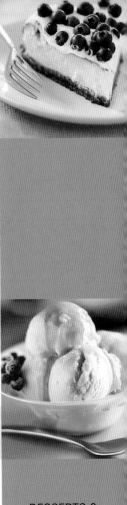

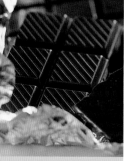

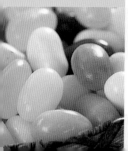

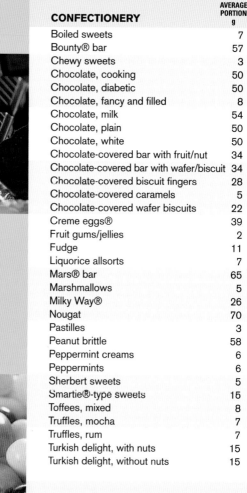

CONFECTIONERY	AVERAGE PORTION g
Boiled sweets	7
Bounty® bar	57
Chewy sweets	3
Chocolate, cooking	50
Chocolate, diabetic	50
Chocolate, fancy and filled	8
Chocolate, milk	54
Chocolate, plain	50
Chocolate, white	50
Chocolate-covered bar with fruit/nut	34
Chocolate-covered bar with wafer/biscuit	34
Chocolate-covered biscuit fingers	28
Chocolate-covered caramels	5
Chocolate-covered wafer biscuits	22
Creme eggs®	39
Fruit gums/jellies	2
Fudge	11
Liquorice allsorts	7
Mars® bar	65
Marshmallows	5
Milky Way®	26
Nougat	70
Pastilles	3
Peanut brittle	58
Peppermint creams	6
Peppermints	6
Sherbert sweets	5
Smartie®-type sweets	15
Toffees, mixed	8
Truffles, mocha	7
Truffles, rum	7
Turkish delight, with nuts	15
Turkish delight, without nuts	15

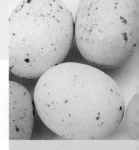

ENERGY kcal	ENERGY kJ	FAT g	SATURATED FAT g	PROTEIN g	CARBOHYDRATE g	FIBRE g
23	98	Trace	0	Trace	6	0
270	1129	15	12.1	3	33	1.4
11	48	1	0.1	0	3	0
275	1147	17	14	2	29	0.6
224	934	15	9.1	5	19	0.6
36	150	2	0.9	0	5	0.1
281	1176	17	9.9	4	31	0.4
255	1069	14	8.4	3	32	1.3
265	1106	15	9.2	4	29	0
170	711	9	4.6	3	20	1.3
170	711	9	4.6	3	20	1.3
134	564	7	3.4	2	18	0.3
23	98	1	0.5	0	3	0
110	462	6	3.8	2	14	0.2
163	681	6	1.8	2	28	0.5
6	28	0	0	0	2	Trace
49	205	2	1	0	9	0
24	104	1	0.3	0	5	0.1
287	1204	12	6.5	3	43	0.7
16	70	0	0	0	4	0
103	435	4	2.2	1	16	0.2
269	1138	6	0.8	3	54	0.6
8	32	0	0	0	2	0
280	1178	11	3.1	5	43	1.2
22	95	Trace	0	0	6	Trace
24	101	0	0	0	6	0
18	76	0	0	0	5	Trace
68	288	3	1.6	1	11	0.2
34	143	1	0.8	0	5	0
34	143	2	1.1	0	4	0.1
36	152	2	1.4	0	3	0.1
52	219	0	0	1	12	0
44	189	0	0	0	12	0

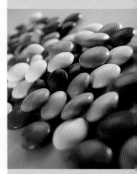

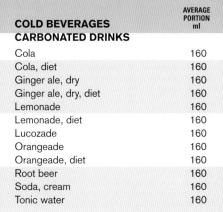

COLD BEVERAGES	AVERAGE PORTION ml
CARBONATED DRINKS	
Cola	160
Cola, diet	160
Ginger ale, dry	160
Ginger ale, dry, diet	160
Lemonade	160
Lemonade, diet	160
Lucozade	160
Orangeade	160
Orangeade, diet	160
Root beer	160
Soda, cream	160
Tonic water	160
FRUIT JUICES	
Apple, unsweetened	160
Carrot	160
Grape, unsweetened	160
Grapefruit, unsweetened	160
Lemon, fresh	10
Lime, fresh	10
Mango, canned	160
Orange, freshly squeezed	160
Orange, unsweetened	160
Passion fruit	160
Pineapple, unsweetened	160
Pomegranate, fresh	160
Prune	160
Tomato	160

ENERGY kcal	ENERGY kJ	FAT g	SATURATED FAT g	PROTEIN g	CARBOHYDRATE g	FIBRE g
66	278	0	0	Trace	17	0
Trace	Trace	0	0	0	0	0
24	99	0	0	0	6	0
2	6	0	0	0	0.4	0
35	149	0	0	Trace	9	0
Trace	Trace	0	0	0	0	0
96	410	0	0	Trace	26	0
113	474	0	0	0	27	0
1	4	0	0	0	0.4	0
66	275	0	0	0	17	0
82	344	0	0	0	21	0
53	226	0	0	0	14	0
61	262	Trace	Trace	0	16	Trace
38	165	Trace	Trace	1	9	0.2
74	314	Trace	Trace	0	19	0
53	224	Trace	Trace	1	13	Trace
1	3	Trace	Trace	0	0	0
1	4	Trace	Trace	0	0	0
62	266	Trace	Trace	0	16	Trace
53	224	Trace	Trace	1	13	0.2
58	245	Trace	Trace	1	14	0.2
75	302	Trace	Trace	1	17	Trace
66	283	Trace	Trace	0	17	Trace
70	302	Trace	Trace	0	19	Trace
91	389	Trace	Trace	1	23	Trace
22	99	Trace	Trace	1	5	1

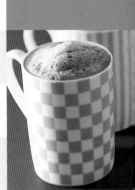

BEVERAGES 133

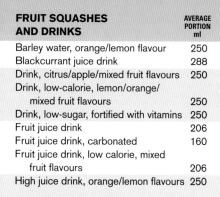

FRUIT SQUASHES AND DRINKS

	AVERAGE PORTION ml
Barley water, orange/lemon flavour	250
Blackcurrant juice drink	288
Drink, citrus/apple/mixed fruit flavours	250
Drink, low-calorie, lemon/orange/ mixed fruit flavours	250
Drink, low-sugar, fortified with vitamins	250
Fruit juice drink	206
Fruit juice drink, carbonated	160
Fruit juice drink, low calorie, mixed fruit flavours	206
High juice drink, orange/lemon flavours	250

MILK-BASED DRINKS

Drinking yogurt	200
Flavoured milk	214
Milkshake, with semi-skimmed milk	300
Milkshake, with skimmed milk	300
Milkshake, with whole milk	300
Milkshake syrup, with semi- skimmed milk	290
Milkshake syrup, with skimmed milk	290
Milkshake syrup, with whole milk	297
Soya milk, flavoured	146
Probiotic yoghurt drink, orange	100
Probiotic yoghurt drink, plain	100

HOT BEVERAGES

Cappuccino, with semi-skimmed milk	190
Cappuccino, with skimmed milk	190
Cappuccino, with whole milk	190
Cocoa, with semi-skimmed milk	250
Cocoa, with skimmed milk	250

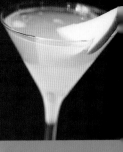

ENERGY kcal	ENERGY kJ	FAT g	SATURATED FAT g	PROTEIN g	CARBOHYDRATE g	FIBRE g
35	150	0	0	0	9	0
86	372	0	0	Trace	23	0
48	200	0	0	Trace	13	0
3	8	0	0	Trace	1	0
10	43	0	0	Trace	3	0
76	328	Trace	Trace	0	20	Trace
62	264	Trace	Trace	Trace	16	Trace
21	89	Trace	Trace	0	5	Trace
63	268	0	0	0	16	0
124	526	Trace	Trace	6	26	Trace
146	614	3	1.9	8	23	0
207	882	5	3	10	34	Trace
171	726	1	0.3	10	34	0
261	1104	11	7.2	9	33	Trace
171	725	4	2.6	8	27	0
136	576	1	0.2	9	27	0
223	936	10	6.2	8	27	0
58	245	2	0.3	4	5	Trace
67	279	0.9	0.6	1.5	13.4	1.3
68	284	1	0.7	1.7	13.1	1.4
46	193	2	1	3	5	0
33	141	0	0.1	3	5	0
65	269	4	2.3	3	5	0
143	608	5	3	9	18	0.5
110	475	1	0.8	9	18	0.5

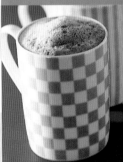

HOT DRINKS	AVERAGE PORTION ml
Cocoa, with whole milk	250
Coffee and chicory essence, with water	190
Coffee, filter	190
Coffee, filter, with semi-skimmed milk	190
Coffee, filter, with skimmed milk	190
Coffee, filter, with single cream	190
Coffee, filter, with whole milk	190
Coffee, instant	190
Coffee, instant, with semi-skimmed milk	190
Coffee, instant, with skimmed milk	190
Coffee, instant, with whole milk	190
Coffee, Irish	125
Drinking chocolate, with semi-skimmed milk	190
Drinking chocolate, with skimmed milk	190
Drinking chocolate, with whole milk	190
Latte, with semi-skimmed milk	190
Latte, with skimmed milk	190
Latte, with whole milk	190
Mocha with semi-skimmed milk	190
Mocha with skimmed milk	190
Mocha with whole milk	190
Ovaltine, with semi-skimmed milk	190
Ovaltine, with skimmed milk	190
Ovaltine, with whole milk	190
Tea, black	190
Tea, Chinese	190
Tea, green	190
Tea, herbal	190
Tea, lemon, instant	190
Tea, with semi-skimmed milk	190
Tea with skimmed milk	190
Tea with whole milk	190

ENERGY kcal	ENERGY kJ	FAT g	SATURATED FAT g	PROTEIN g	CARBOHYDRATE g	FIBRE g
190	800	10	6.5	9	17	0.5
17	76	Trace	0	0	5	0
4	15	Trace	Trace	0	1	0
13	55	1	0.2	1	1	0
11	43	0	0	1	1	0
27	106	2	1.3	1	1	0
13	59	1	0.6	1	1	0
Trace	4	Trace	0	0	Trace	0
13	55	1	0.2	1	1	0
8	39	0	0	1	1	0
15	65	1	0.6	1	1	0
105	433	10	6.1	1	4	0
135	578	4	2.3	7	21	Trace
112	481	1	0.6	7	21	Trace
171	716	8	4.8	6	20	Trace
60	252	2	1.3	4	7	0
33	141	1	0.1	3	5	0
85	353	5	3	4	6	0
96	405	5	3.1	4	9	0.1
81	339	3	2	4	9	0.1
120	500	7	4.8	4	9	0.1
150	642	3	1.9	7	25	Trace
129	549	1	0.2	7	25	Trace
184	779	7	4.6	7	25	Trace
Trace	4	Trace	Trace	0	Trace	0
2	10	0	0	0	0	0
Trace	Trace	0	0	0	Trace	0
2	25	Trace	Trace	0	0	0
15	65	0	0	0	4	0
13	53	1	0.2	1	1	0
8	36	0	0	1	1	0
15	61	1	0.6	1	1	0

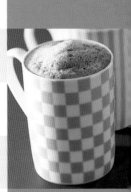

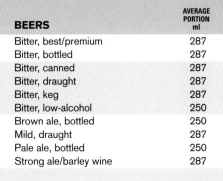

BEERS	AVERAGE PORTION ml
Bitter, best/premium	287
Bitter, bottled	287
Bitter, canned	287
Bitter, draught	287
Bitter, keg	287
Bitter, low-alcohol	250
Brown ale, bottled	250
Mild, draught	287
Pale ale, bottled	250
Strong ale/barley wine	287

CIDERS	
Dry	287
Low-alcohol	250
Sweet	287
Vintage	287

LAGERS	
Bottled	250
Canned	287
Draught	287
Low-alcohol	250
Premium	287
Shandy	287

ENERGY kcal	ENERGY kJ	FAT g	SATURATED FAT g	PROTEIN g	CARBOHYDRATE g	FIBRE g
95	399	Trace	Trace	1	6	Trace
86	356	Trace	Trace	1	6	Trace
92	379	Trace	Trace	1	7	0
92	379	Trace	Trace	1	7	0
89	370	Trace	Trace	1	7	0
33	135	0	0	1	5	Trace
75	315	Trace	Trace	1	8	Trace
69	293	Trace	Trace	1	5	Trace
70	295	Trace	Trace	1	5	Trace
189	789	Trace	Trace	2	18	Trace
103	436	0	0	Trace	7	0
43	185	0	0	Trace	9	0
121	505	0	0	Trace	12	0
290	1208	0	0	Trace	21	0
73	300	Trace	Trace	1	4	0
83	347	Trace	Trace	1	Trace	Trace
83	347	Trace	Trace	1	Trace	Trace
25	103	Trace	Trace	1	4	Trace
169	700	Trace	Trace	1	7	Trace
32	138	0	0	Trace	9	Trace

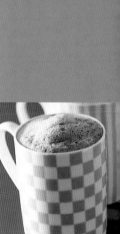

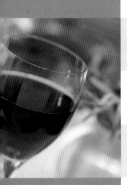

LIQUEURS	AVERAGE PORTION ml
Advocaat	25
Cherry Brandy	25
Coîntreau	25
Cream liqueurs	25
Crème de Menthe	25
Curaçao	25
Drambuie	25
Egg nog	160
Grand Marnier	25
Pernod	25
Southern Comfort	25
Tia Maria	25

FORTIFIED WINES	
Port	50
Sherry, dry	50
Sherry, medium	50
Sherry, sweet	50
Tonic wine	125
Vermouth, dry	48
Vermouth, sweet	48

SPIRITS, 40% VOLUME	
Brandy	25
Gin	25
Rum	25
Vodka	25
Whisky	25

ENERGY kcal	ENERGY kJ	FAT g	SATURATED FAT g	PROTEIN g	CARBOHYDRATE g	FIBRE g
65	273	2	0.5	1	7	0
66	275	0	0	Trace	8	0
79	328	0	0	Trace	6	0
81	338	4	0	Trace	6	0
66	275	0	0	Trace	8	0
78	326	0	0	Trace	7	0
79	328	0	0	Trace	6	0
182	763	7	3.4	6	16	0
79	328	0	0	Trace	6	0
79	328	0	0	Trace	6	0
79	328	0	0	Trace	6	0
66	275	0	0	Trace	8	0
79	328	0	0	0	6	0
58	241	0	0	0	1	0
58	241	0	0	0	3	0
68	284	0	0	0	3	0
159	665	0	0	Trace	15	0
52	217	0	0	0	1	0
72	303	0	0	Trace	8	0
52	215	0	0	Trace	Trace	0
52	215	0	0	Trace	Trace	0
52	215	0	0	Trace	Trace	0
52	215	0	0	Trace	Trace	0
52	215	0	0	Trace	Trace	0

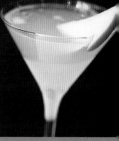

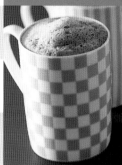

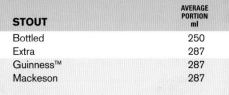

STOUT	AVERAGE PORTION ml
Bottled	250
Extra	287
Guinness™	287
Mackeson	287

WINES	
Champagne	125
Mulled wine	125
Red wine	125
Rosé, medium	125
White wine, dry	125
White wine, medium	125
White wine, sparkling	125
White wine, sweet	125

ENERGY kcal	ENERGY kJ	FAT g	SATURATED FAT g	PROTEIN g	CARBOHYDRATE g	FIBRE g
93	390	Trace	Trace	1	10	0
112	468	Trace	Trace	1	6	0
86	362	Trace	Trace	1	4	0
103	439	Trace	Trace	1	13	0
95	394	0	0	0	2	0
245	1028	0	0	0	32	0
85	354	0	0	0	0	0
89	368	0	0	0	3	0
83	344	0	0	0	1	0
93	385	0	0	0	4	0
93	384	0	0	0	6	0
118	493	0	0	0	7	0

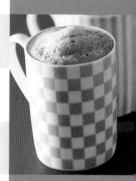

© **Burger King** 66–67.
Octopus Publishing Group Limited 123 top right, /Jean Cazals 71 bottom right, 132 top left, /Stephen Conroy 101 top right, 127 bottom right, 130 bottom left, 131 top right, /Gus Filgate 52 bottom left, /Jeremy Hopley 8 top left, 59 bottom right, 132 bottom left, /David Jordan 8 bottom left, 16 top left, 58 bottom left, 76 bottom left, 77 top right, 87 top right, 102 bottom left, 131 bottom right, 133 bottom right, /Graham Kirk 126 bottom left, /Sandra Lane 86 bottom left, 114 bottom left, /William Lingwood 16 bottom left, 17 top right, 17 bottom right, 71 top right, 76 top left, 77 bottom right, 99 bottom right, 103 bottom right, 109 top right, /Neil Mersh 58 top left, 59 top left, /Peter Myers 52 top left, 130 top left, /Sean Myers 70 top left, 70 bottom left, /William Reavell 34 top left, 34 bottom left, 35 top right, 53 top right, 53 bottom right, 80 bottom left, 94 top left, 95 top right, 98 top left, 100 top left, 100 bottom left, 101 bottom right, 106 top left, 106 bottom left, 107 bottom right, 108 top left, 108 bottom left, 114 top left, 115 top right, 126 top left, 127 top right, 133 top right, /Simon Smith 80 top left, 81 top right, 81 bottom right, 95 bottom right, 102 top left, 103 top right, 107 top right, 122 top left, 122 bottom left, /Ian Wallace 9 top right, 9 bottom right, 86 top left, 87 bottom right, 94 bottom left, 99 top right, 109 bottom right, 115 bottom right, /Philip Webb 35 bottom right, 98 bottom left, 123 bottom right.
© **Kentucky Fried Chicken** 68–69.

Commissioning Editor Nicola Hill
Editorial Director Jane Birch
Copy Editor Cathy Lowne
Executive Art Editor Rozelle Bentheim
Designer Peter Gerrish
Picture Researchers Zoe Holtermann, Jennifer Veall
Production Controller Lucy Woodhead